Your HEALTH, Your DECISIONS

Your HEALTH, Your DECISIONS

HOW TO WORK WITH YOUR DOCTOR TO

BECOME A KNOWLEDGE-POWERED PATIENT

ROBERT ALAN McNUTT, M.D.

THE UNIVERSITY OF NORTH CAROLINA PRESS *Chapel Hill*

Designed by Richard Hendel
Set in Utopia and Aller types
by codeMantra
Manufactured in the United States of America

The University of North Carolina Press has been a
member of the Green Press Initiative since 2003.

Jacket illustration: © stevecoleimages; iStockphoto.com

Library of Congress Cataloging-in-Publication Data
Names: McNutt, Robert Alan, author.
Title: Your health, your decisions : how to work with your doctor to
become a knowledge-powered patient / Robert Alan McNutt.
Description: Chapel Hill : The University of North Carolina Press, [2016] |
Includes bibliographical references and index.
Identifiers: LCCN 2016004008 |
ISBN 9781469629179 (cloth : alk. paper) | ISBN 9781469629186 (ebook)
Subjects: LCSH: Medical care—Decision making. | Physician and patient.
Classification: LCC R723.5 .M36 2016 | DDC 610.69/6—dc23
LC record available at http://lccn.loc.gov/2016004008

Contents

Tables and Figures

Tables

Figures

Preface

My name is Robert McNutt. I graduated from Michigan State University (MSU) in 1971 with a bachelor's degree in Arts and Humanities. My plan was to be a high school teacher and swimming coach. But, as a wise saying reminds us, life is what happens while making plans—while on the path to becoming a teacher I decided to apply to medical school. The application process required me to test my ability to intellectually survive medical training. The medical school application test and I did not get along well: my score was low, since there were few questions on the test about philosophy or the humanities. Despite this, however, I was granted an interview for admission at MSU.

The interviewing professor, a psychiatrist, held two pieces of paper, one in each hand, and glanced back and forth at them. After a moment, he asked me how my grades in the humanities—Phi Beta Kappa level—could be reconciled with what, he said, was a low medical school admission score. Our ensuing discussion lasted over an hour. I said that the test did not ask questions I expected based on my understanding of what it meant to be a physician, which derived from experiences in my home. I said that my grandparents and several uncles died in our home with my family caring for them. I told the interviewer how important a doctor was to our family and how much we appreciated help when we were ill, and also how much we appreciated kindness at the limits of the physician's expertise. I told him I still remembered a physician's visit to our home for my ill sister, and that my dad and the physician shared whiskey after the work was done. I said I wanted to go into medicine to share a metaphoric (perhaps, occasionally, literal) whiskey with each person I would be privileged to care for.

Apparently, the professor liked whiskey—I was accepted into MSU's medical school, and thankfully, the medical admission test score did not predict my success. After graduating in 1975, I did my internship in general/family medicine, worked in an emergency room in rural Michigan, and then returned for internal medicine training and, finally, training in oncology. After my fellowship in oncology and hematology, I practiced in a solo and, later, a two-person oncology practice.

During my private practice years, I saw medicine's goals and actions drastically change. Information was being produced in vast quantities; patients were being reassigned diagnostic labels; treatments were propagating. I saw the rise of uncertainty in benefits and harms inherent in our burgeoning numbers of tests and treatments. I read studies in cancer care showing advances, but the advances did not seem to extend to my or my colleagues' patients. I watched the medical system embrace technology at the expense of philosophy. I saw patients being packaged into averages rather than being valued as individuals. As a result of my observations, I decided to learn the methods of science to better answer questions posed by my patients, and to reconcile discrepancies between what I read and what I observed while caring for patients.

So, I went back to school in the early 1990s with a National Library of Medicine fellowship at Tufts New England Medical Center and attended classes to learn epidemiology, statistics, and decision analysis. After three years of additional training, I returned to practice as an academic physician. The University of North Carolina at Chapel Hill, the University of Wisconsin, Chicago's John H. Stroger Jr. Hospital of Cook County, and Rush University Medical Center have been my academic homes.

During the academic years I experienced nearly every medical task, from clinician to researcher. I obtained grant funds from a range of agencies, including the National Institutes of Health (NIH); I wrote over two hundred papers and abstracts and presented my research at national meetings; I ran a medical clinic; I became the medical director of an HMO (health maintenance organization), chairman of internal medicine at a medical school, director of a health services research unit, director of research at a safety-net hospital, and director of a program in patient safety research. I was a member of national committees, ran national programs for the Society of Medical Decision Making, and reviewed grant applications for the NIH and the Veterans Administration. I was interviewed to be on the Center for Medicare and Medicaid Services governing board; I became an editor or board member at three journals most recently at the *Journal of the American Medical Association.*

Being an editor and researcher has allowed me to observe and conduct nearly every type of study on numerous topics in medicine, and I have learned how information can mislead to the ultimate detriment of a patient's care. I also noticed, as mentioned above, that, philosophically, the medical system was abdicating its responsibility to individuals in order to support a science of populations. But populations get better only by improving care for individuals. Unfortunately, in my view, medical leaders have become too interested in the medical system for its own sake, and the way we now conduct science supports systems rather than individual patients. Science will be better when it is conducted in such a way that it supports individuals' rights to participate in their own medical care. Presently, medical care is a top-down industry (medical business on the top directing decisions down to patients)—we must reorient to a profession that puts the patient on top. Medicine will emerge as a truly successful profession only if it aligns exclusively with patients' rights and abilities to fully contribute to their care.

And, my experiences tell me that it is important for each of us, as patients, to now fully participate in our own care. The production of good and bad information is escalating. Learning what information is reliable and then learning how to use that information to enhance our medical choices have become indispensable skills for a healthy life. However, fully contributing to medical decisions requires training in medical decision making—wanting to be involved in care is not enough. But rest assured, making sound medical choices is a skill that can be learned by almost anyone. My aim in this book is to provide you with a simple method to learn these essential skills so that you can find and understand reliable medical information, weigh your testing and treatment options, and make sound choices to direct your medical future.

———

It is a difficult task to acknowledge all those who have meant so much to me during my career in medicine. Foremost, I have a wonderful, supportive family, and I appreciated their patience while they listened, over and over, to me express my ideas for this book. Their critical insights and thoughtful additions are woven through the book. I love you all, and you know who you are. My children and grandchildren humble me with their grace. (Les and Craig, your support especially moved me forward.)

Experts in clinical care, research, health policy, editing, and writing have blessed me throughout my medical life. I have stood up for patients alongside the best. I trained in oncology with one of the small number of nationally recognized clinical professors of oncology, Dr. George Suhrland, who is now gone from this world but not from my heart. Drs. Stephen Pauker and Harry Selker pushed me to creative heights while teaching me how to think about science and decision analysis. Dr. Nortin Hadler never lets me off the hook for any idea I might have. Dr. Cathy DeAngelis nurtured me and spurred me to think outside the box as an editor. Dr. Stuart Levin showed me how leadership matters when trying to change the way medical care is practiced for the betterment of patients. There are so many others—truly, I have been blessed.

But, I most appreciate my patients. You are the reason that I went into medicine, and you remain the only reason. You have taught me the most. I am writing this book for you. You deserve your best medical care.

A Road Map of This Book

We are about to begin a journey together. This book will follow a path, albeit a winding one, that shows you how to fully participate in your own medical decisions. The book is as much narrative as exposition. The process that will make you a better medical decision maker is illustrated in stories. This book is my story, my patients' stories, and your story. The better you understand medical decision-making stories, the better you will be at directing your own medical future. I will ask you to believe that you are the main medical decision maker. And as a by-product of your participation, by perfect-storm circumstance, you will contribute to medical care that matters ideally.

Every journey starts with a goal in sight, so here is our itinerary:

In the introduction and the first chapter, I present one of my patient's medical dilemmas as an example of the problems with making medical decisions today.

In the second chapter, I describe my medical decision-making journey and introduce how to make a decision using a checklist based on decision science.

In chapters 3 and 4, I argue that you are the best medical-decision maker and show reasons why.

After discussing why you must fully participate in your decisions, in chapters 5 and 6 you will learn the science behind medical choices and become a better user of medical information.

Next, in chapters 7, 8, and 9 you will practice the skills needed for making medical decisions. These skills show you how to make information work for you.

Then chapters 10 through 16 present stories of patients making decisions. You will be surprised how similar their medical decisions are to yours, and you will learn, like they did, to overcome obstacles to making choices.

Chapter 17 discusses some limits of studies used to inform patients and what to consider if no or conflicting information is present.

Chapter 18 presents some clarifications, gives examples of patients who went to their physicians as informed decision makers, and ponders some of their physicians' responses. In doing so, we will take a critical look at the ideas I have shared with you in the preceding chapters.

Finally, chapter 19 provides useful sources of medical information.

These chapters will walk you through the reasons that you need to make your own medical decisions, some principles and methods you can use to better understand medical information, and techniques you can use to apply that information to your own specific medical encounters. Along the way, I hope to entertain and enlighten you with tales of medical adventures that I have collected in my almost forty years of helping patients live better lives, so that you, too, can be confident enough to make personal, participatory, informed choices and achieve the best medical care.

Your **HEALTH**, Your **DECISIONS**

Introduction

Mrs. D. (not her real initial) set a record: I was her eighth "second-opinion" physician. Until recently Mrs. D. had been healthy—she had never missed a day of work, and her retirement had been a whirlwind of activities. The abruptness of her diagnosis, as much as the diagnosis itself, sent her emotions reeling: in the span of less than a week, a small trickle of blood, then some tests, then finding cancer that would not be cured.

Mrs. D.'s personal physician did not feel equipped to be her treating physician—treating cancer long ago moved out of the generalist's office to offices of physicians trained specifically in the care of patients with cancer—so he sent her to a specialist. We do not know exactly what happened at that specialist's visit, but Mrs. D. and her husband left the encounter dissatisfied. A call to their family physician resulted in a second consultant, who offered a treatment plan and, additionally, said they might want another's opinion because there are other options for care. More consultants followed, a procession propelled in part by physicians and in part by the patient, until she found her way to my office.

When I met Mrs. and Mr. D., they gave me a list of the treatment options proposed by the seven consultants. The options numbered eight; some were conflicting, but some were similar except for nuances. They did a wonderful job, tearfully at times, telling me their tale of seeking the best option for the treatment of her cancer. To them, each option was less than ideal. They were focused on the performance of the treatments and what each would entail. Radiation, surgery, and/or chemotherapy require different efforts to complete: some take weeks, some take days.

They looked exhausted, worn by worry. I said that if they were too tired for more discussion, I would reschedule. They came to life with that suggestion and said, "No! We are eager to get a treatment started." However, their ability to make a decision was frozen by fear and the complexity of sorting through treatment plans. After she had outlined the options and her understanding of them, she asked me what I thought she should do, asking for a ninth option or, at least, a weighing in on the already proposed options. I smiled and said: "Mrs. D., you do not need any more opinions, nor do you need me to pick from the list. You are the one who must make the decision. Offering you a ninth, or even a second, opinion is not a physician's job. His or her job is to help you learn how to make your decision. You must balance and compare the harms and benefits of therapies from your perspective. My role is a partner on your decision-making journey."

I remember, in retrospect, that Mrs. and Mr. D. had puzzled looks on their faces after my comment. I must have noticed their expressions because I then began asking questions to ease their discomfort. I asked her to tell me how each option compared in terms of their abilities to extend her life. She did not know, had not been told, and had not asked. I then asked her to tell me how each option compared in terms of their likelihood of causing harmful side effects. She did not know, had not been told, and had not asked.

1

A Story of Failed Decision Making

Mrs. D.'s tale is a story of failed medical decision making. Unfortunately, other than the number of consultants, it is a usual story: patients visit multiple physicians, who offer different testing or treatment plans. Patients are regularly overwhelmed when bombarded with options for care, and it is common that, despite these visits with physicians, patients do not know how much better or worse the offered tests or treatments are.

"Better" or "worse," however, are imprecise terms. Each disease of mankind disturbs in different ways. Some diseases cause us to suffer symptoms suddenly. Others threaten us slowly over long periods of time. Every disease is associated with outcomes, which are measurable, quantifiable events that are the consequences of both disease conditions and medical tests or treatments. Outcomes can be increased or decreased symptoms (such as pain), better or worse function (such as ability to care for yourself), life or death, and, from a testing standpoint, a correct diagnosis or a missed or false one. When faced with a malady, we seek medical care to diminish untoward events. The goal of medical treatment is, of course, to reduce the chance of adverse outcomes caused by your disease from occurring or, perhaps, to lengthen the time before adverse outcomes eventually occur. However, attempts to treat the disease-related outcomes have a flip side. The flip side is that tests and treatments are not perfect. In most cases, a test or treatment that reduces adverse outcomes of disease increases other adverse outcomes caused by the test or treatment itself. Hence, a trade-off occurs in medical-decision situations: a treatment that offers an added chance of having the best outcomes from the disease standpoint must be balanced against the added chance, simultaneously, that this same treatment may also cause harm in some other way. This contest between good and bad is the normal situation in medical decision making, but it is rarely understood by the patient. In over forty years of medical practice, I have never had a patient who came to me able to recount the absolute differences in outcomes associated with the tests or treatments being contemplated. However, this is also my experience with physicians.

Not knowing the absolute differences in outcomes is the basis of the failed process of medical decision making in Mrs. D.'s story. Her experience exposes mistaken beliefs about the best way to achieve excellent medical care. The failed process includes the beliefs by physicians (a) that they are the ones to offer choices and (b) that decisions, based on medical expertise, are solely theirs to make. These misplaced physician beliefs are supported too often by patients' belief that physicians are experts on what is best for the patient. These beliefs stifle the progress of personal, participatory, informed choice and best medical care.

And Mrs. D.'s story is not unique. Here are other examples of problems faced by my patients—misplaced beliefs play out in each:

A man had a routine exam, and his physician ordered a test for prostate-specific antigen (PSA). The test result was abnormal; cancer was found. The patient was told surgery would cure; surgery was scheduled.

A woman was told her mammogram was abnormal, and she was scheduled for a second, "better" test. That test found even more abnormalities that may or may not be cancer. She was scheduled for a biopsy of some of the abnormal areas and a repeat test.

A woman with a numb arm was asked to have a "stress test" to make sure that heart disease was not missed. After the first test result, she was told other tests were needed. She was scheduled for two more tests.

A man who had smoked his entire life was asked to have a computerized axial tomography (CAT) scan to find cancer early should it be there. The scan was scheduled.

A woman taking a single medicine to protect from a stroke was told to take a second to further safeguard her. A prescription for the new medicine ended her visit.

A physician asked a woman recently diagnosed with ductal carcinoma in situ (DCIS) in one breast if she wanted a bilateral mastectomy (both breasts removed). The patient said yes, and the physician scheduled surgery.

Each of these patients had a choice in every circumstance. In most medical care situations, multiple options are available, which differ on the amount of benefit and harm they may produce. The patients described above later made different choices for their care than the ones originally proposed and scheduled by their physicians (we will read about some of these decision processes later in the book). Each patient stopped for a moment and asked for more information. Each, after reflecting on the added information with their physicians, changed course: the surgery for prostate cancer was canceled, as was the breast biopsy; multiple tests were canceled after the first one; the prescription for the new medicine was thrown away; the CAT scan to screen for lung cancer was canceled, as was the bilateral mastectomy.

It is common that patients chose differently after being informed. Choosing differently does not mean they always select fewer tests or forgo treatments; sometimes they choose more tests and more aggressive treatments. The tests or treatments that patients choose after being informed depend on their values, and that means peoples' choices will vary. That is the point, and the goal. The patients described above learned to make their own decisions. They learned the evidence about the potential for benefit and harm for each choice and decided based on their unique clinical circumstances in light of the evidence. This is the goal of medical care: patient choice based on personal preferences for the chances of added benefit and harm afforded by one treatment versus another. This sort of personal, variable, individualistic medical decision making is the core of an ethical, value-laden medical care system.

To make these educated decisions about your own medical care, you must understand more clearly how modern medicine is practiced today. This includes knowing more about how treatments come to be offered in the medical marketplace. You must also know whether the evidence from medical experiments is useful for you. You are about to learn that just because a study of a test or treatment has been done and the results published in a medical journal does not mean that it is useful information, or even true. You will need to know if information about treatments is correct and, if so, whether it is pertinent to you.

Last, you must know how to use the best medical evidence available to be able to fully participate in your own medical decisions.

Mrs. D. and her husband learned the process of medical decision making. They learned the added chances of harms and benefits of the proposed treatment plans. They struggled with the choice, because there was no easy way out. Mrs. D eventually made a choice based on her preferences. What Mrs. and Mr. D. learned is yours to learn as well—this book will give you the tools you need to meaningfully evaluate options proposed to you. The chapters that follow present a commonsense set of steps to follow when you are faced with a medical decision. The steps will lead you to a deliberate and coherent decision-making process.

You may be asking, why learn to make choices if physicians make them? There are compelling reasons for you to be a full participant in your own medical decisions. Before discussing the process of medical decision making and watching patients decide, I summarize these reasons. I will show you that physicians are not as well trained as you think to make medical decisions for you—they need your help.

2

My Medical-Decision-Making Story

In the preface I introduced myself. Here I give a little more of my background. I want you to know enough about me so that you can judge my qualifications as a guide to help you make medical decisions, and to suggest to you that I have an uncommon amount of experience for understanding the value of medical studies and how information can be misleading. I am also one of only one hundred or so physicians in the United States trained formally in medical decision making, from both a health policy and an individual patient perspective.

But, I don't want you to think for even a moment that I am a special medical decision maker or, in fact, special in any way. My experiences serve only to prepare me to help you—you are the special person in medical care. I am writing this book so you can have the tools to advocate for your best medical care. I still embrace the premise that medicine should not be a business but a profession; a profession solely serves the patient's best interests without other considerations.

So, despite my experiences in medical care, I do not want to, and will not be able to, make decisions for you. No physician can, or should. I suppose one of my motives in describing myself is for you to see that if this physician, with all his experience and training in medical care and research and decision science, can't make decisions for you, then no one will be able to decide but you. It is my hope that you come to believe that you need to fully participate in your own medical decisions.

While I entered medical school with the belief that only patients should make medical decisions, acting on this belief was easier said than done. It was difficult because the medical training program did not share my belief. The medical school environment and my teachers were reluctant to place decisions in the hands of patients. Many said patients would not be able to make decisions, because they have no training in medicine, so trained physicians must help. But it may surprise you to learn that few medical schools train physicians in explicit ways to make medical decisions—as if learning how to make decisions is supposed to seep into a medical student's consciousness.

Thankfully, my teachers' views about how decisions should be meted out did not discourage me. It was obvious to me: the patient should decide. (Of course, sometimes this is not possible. For example, I have never asked patients to decide if they wanted a blood transfusion if they were bleeding seriously from an injury, or asked them if they wanted fluids if they were in shock. Urgent care requires urgent, trained choices. But these urgent decisions are not the norm. Most often patients have chronic, slow-moving diseases that allow time to make decisions.) So, teachers aside, what did patients say about being their own medical decision maker? The patients would see it my way, for sure, even if my professors did not.

But I was distressed to find that patients, too, often disagreed with me—many expected me to make choices for them. One of my patients responded, when I asked for his preference for treatment, "How should I know? You're the doctor." However, making a decision is a personal act. It may be the only act under our own control. Whom we love, what we do with our time, what we eat—these are our choices to make. For each aspect of our daily life, we choose among alternatives. Our personalities are, in part, the accumulation of the personal choices we make. The decisions we make do not become mere entries in a diary. Instead, these decisions, their consequences, and our responses to those consequences make us who we are. Our choices become our personal histories. This is especially true for medical decisions.

Since medical decision making requires choosing, we might assume that a science of choice would be taught during training. Since medicine is a science, I expected to learn in medical school as much about the science of making decisions as I would learn about biology, physiology, and anatomy. I was mistaken—I spent hours hunched over books on physiology and biology, but I never had to study how to make a decision. When I asked my professors to teach me how to make a decision, they said, "Learn by experience."

Their method for learning how to make a medical decision (the experience of watching others decide) sounded similar to how I was told to make decisions in my personal life. Even my loving, logical parents would turn to "experience" to support their arguments about what their contentious son should and should not do. Experience, as a decision-making tool, did not ring true to either a rebellious teen or a budding physician—it simply could not be the best way to help patients with their complex decisions. Sure, I would get experience by watching and learning, but how would I translate experience with one patient to another? And what if my experiences were unusual? Insufficient?

The only way I was going to be comfortable with informing patients was to be comfortable with how we went about making a decision together. This is because, no matter how good a decision is, the consequences of a decision are out of our control. Just because a better-for-you treatment is chosen does not mean that the results will be good. And conversely, it does not mean you decided correctly if, after you choose, you have a good outcome. Chance plays out after a choice, but making the choice should not be left to chance. Given this fact, the goal is to follow a process that balances the potential good and bad outcomes that may result from choosing one test or treatment over another, *before* you make the choice.

With medical school failing to show me a method for helping patients make choices, I sought advice from others who were practiced with decisions. I asked financial counselors, CEOs, psychologists, scientists, clergy, parents, and even (for fun) a palm reader. Here are some of the more humorous responses to my queries:

"Do the right thing." (palm reader)
"Use your gut instinct." (gastroenterologist, scientist)
"Put your decisions in the hands of a higher power." (financial
    counselor, pointing to her book on playing the stock market)
"Ultimately, the best decision maker must be the one who decides."
    (CEO)
"Weigh the risk and the benefit." (father)
"Quit worrying so much." (mother, psychologist)
"Get advice from the expert." (clergy)

These decision-making experts espoused a consistent theme: decision making was an art of experience and emotion, not a science or a "method." But decision making is not an art, because the value of art is in the eyes of the beholder. Medical care cannot be a profession of different "eyes of the beholder" when it is the physicians' eyes doing the beholding. It can be a profession only if it is a science and, additionally, if patients are providing the worth of the scientific art.

Thankfully, there *is* a science of medical decision making. I learned this science during a fellowship that taught how to use decision science with individual people and with decision makers interested in health policy. That science, called decision analysis, provides the best framework to help individuals make decisions.

Using decision analysis to choose among options has several benefits that enable sound choices. The primary advantages are:

- First, it requires you to rigorously study options (more than one test or treatment).
- Second, it requires you to compare these options. Comparing reveals the absolute differences in outcomes imposed by the varied options: the number or percentage of patients having critical outcomes caused by the disease, or caused by the test or treatment. In fact, medical decision making requires choosing among treatments that often differ more by the inch than by the mile. Improved chances of better outcomes for the disease have to be balanced with additional chances of worse outcomes from the test or treatment, and usually these chances are small differences on both sides of the equation. You should not think of medical treatments as cure-alls. Medical care is usually doled out in steps, not leaps and bounds, and you must decide for each step whether it makes the trip worthwhile.
- Third, decision analysis requires you to incorporate your personality and preferences into the decision. It is you who decides whether the absolute differences in benefit are worth the absolute differences in harm.

Based on these ideas, I developed a process for medical decision making with patients. The process is grounded in information about how much more benefit and how much more harm you might expect by choosing one test or treatment rather than another. The method, after showing the scientific information, requires and allows you to use your own feelings about the differences in the outcomes of care as the way to balance the trade-off between more benefit and more harm, which medical care often involves. Few tests or treatments provide only beneficial outcomes. It is the nature of medical science that, as we advance, our treatments add complications. There is no way out of this predicament, and this is precisely why *you* must be the medical decision maker.

I have used the process of medical decision making outlined in this book for over twenty-five years. I have refined the process by working with patients who had to make decisions. I know the process will help you. The steps involved, a kind of checklist, are outlined below. Please don't be daunted—we will study and practice each step until they are familiar to you. By going step by step, you will learn the skills of medical decision making.

DECISION-MAKING CHECKLIST

1. Slow down: take time to decide. Don't let fear dictate your choice.
2. Slow down: take time to decide. Don't let fear dictate your choice. (repeated on purpose)
3. Know your diagnosis. Diseases differ even if they carry the same name.
4. Study the experiments that test options for your care. Determine, for all options, what number and percentage of people in the study had the outcomes—both good and bad.
   a. Determine the percentage of people who had the outcome caused by disease for each treatment.
   b. Subtract the percentages of people having the outcome caused by the disease for compared options. This difference is the added chance of benefit.
   c. Determine the percentage of people who had the outcome caused by treatment for compared options.
   d. Subtract the percentages of people having the outcome caused by the treatment for compared options. This difference is the added chance of harm.
5. Compare the difference in the added chances of benefit and harm; use graphics to help you understand.
6. Assess your unique clinical situation, and modify the numbers for your situation.
7. Determine if the added chance of benefit afforded by one treatment compared with another is worth the added chance of harm caused by that same treatment compared with the other.
8. If you are not clear what to do, repeat steps 1 through 8.

3

Why Not Just Ask My Doctor What to Do?

The title of this chapter invites a challenge—aimed at me. I already noted what my teachers in medical school thought about who should make medical decisions: physicians. Were they wrong? Yes. Should, and can, patients participate fully in their decisions? Yes—my patients do it all the time. You will soon see that you can learn how to make medical choices. But there are equally compelling reasons why you not only can but *must* fully participate in your medical decisions. It is not in your best interest to follow solely another's advice. Medical care is about what *you* want, not what others think you might or should want.

The most critical of the compelling reasons to become more involved in your care follow and are discussed in depth further below.

1. You are the one who faces the consequences of your choice (foremost reason).
2. Physicians too often offer and advocate for a single option for care.
3. Physicians do not adequately communicate the consequences of the options compared.
4. Physicians are not ideally trained to make decisions with individuals because nowadays they are trained to decide for "average" populations.
5. Regrettably, financial conflicts of interests may lead physicians to propose tests or treatments that are not in your best interest.
6. Regrettably, fear of lawsuits may also lead physicians to propose tests or treatments that are not in your best interest.

Reason 1: You Are the One Who Faces the Consequences of Your Choice

In a 2004 editorial in the *Journal of the American Medical Association* (*JAMA*), I wrote that patients and physicians could not share medical decisions.[1] The concept of sharing is readily understood if there are joint interests. For example, my grandkids can share toys: one plays with the toy for a time, and then the other takes a turn. My kids can share food, because food can be divided and each may imbibe. Sharing is the *combined* ownership of the events or items being shared.

Medical decision making, however, has no notion of sharing. Since there is no joint ownership of the outcomes of your choice of a diagnostic test or a treatment for your malady, you must make sure a decision is best for you, on your terms. No physician, family member, adviser, insurer, or government can know how you would feel about the potential outcomes you may face when you are ill—I never suffered the side effects of the chemotherapy I prescribed; my patients did. Hence, only they should decide if the chemotherapy's potential to add to their life is worth the complications they will suffer.

I claim that the term used for the concept of patients being involved in medical decision making should be "informed medical decision making" rather than "shared medical decision making." Words shape concepts and are the building blocks of understanding, and the only concept that matters is that you must participate fully in your medical choices after being informed. The term "shared medical decision making" persists, but sharing decisions is impossible. Since only patients face the consequences of medical choices, they should be the primary decision makers.

Reason 2: Physicians Don't Allow You to Make Choices Because They Pronounce and Advocate for Choices

Let's set up an ideal situation to introduce this topic. You have a complaint; you go to a physician; a diagnosis is made; a discussion follows that allows you to decide among competing treatment options based on your feelings about how much better and how much worse one treatment is versus another. This is the goal, but is it the usual situation?

I had an opportunity to watch videotapes of physicians and their patients during visits in the physicians' offices. These videotapes, conducted with the consent of both the physicians and the patients, were part of a program to test different methods to evaluate physicians trained in internal medicine (which encompasses all of the medical fields except for surgery, obstetrics, and pediatrics). Residents, prior to being deemed eligible for the medical board exam, learn their craft in a series of rotations (intensive care, general medicine, cardiology, etc.), usually experienced on a monthly basis, and each rotation requires a passing grade but not an exam. The pass/fail assessments are surprisingly subjective, despite some broad criteria, such as "professionalism" or "knowledge," guiding the evaluation.

The residents being videotaped were in their last year of internal medicine training and were about to enter practice. This direct examination of their actions allowed us to evaluate, among other things, how they interacted with patients. Both the physicians and the patients knew they were being videotaped and that the videotape would be used as part of an evaluation. This sort of anxiety-provoking exercise would, we expected, alert the physicians to be on their toes and to perform their best.

As part of this exam, the physicians had to discuss a decision with the patient. The decisions most often involved ordering a test (such as getting a chest x-ray to check for pneumonia for a patient with a cough) or starting a medicine. For treatment options, such as medicines, we expected physicians would tell patients about options (for example, "We have two medicines we could use") and then compare one medicine versus another (for example, "Both of these medicines lower blood pressure equally, but one is less expensive and has 10 percent fewer side effects"). But this is not what I observed—physicians did not compare options for patients by providing benefit and harm differences, not even in general terms, much less in terms of the numeric differences in the chances of the outcomes the patient may face. Not once did I see a trade-off discussed. What did I see instead? Most announced a single decision ("I am going to start this medicine . . ."), followed by a reason for the decision ("because this medicine will protect your kidneys").

A concern about my recounting of these videotaped encounters is, perhaps, that my expectations were too high for what should happen during a patient-physician encounter. After all, each of the residents eventually passed the training program and went to practice, and these physicians were trainees at the time the videotapes were done and not fully in practice, even though their three-year training in internal medicine was nearly complete. So these videos may not have represented the usual practice of medical care. But who trained these trainees? Teaching physicians, who were the trainees' role models, that's who. If these teachers had taught informed communication, and if they had expected a patient-decision model to be used, I should have seen informed, patient-involved decisions during these evaluations. But I didn't. If these videotapes even remotely capture usual practice, informed patients making decisions is not the norm.

Mrs. D. might agree with my observations. She saw seven specialists before coming to my office; all but one had presented a single option, and none told her the differences among options. Mrs. D. and you, like her, cannot assume that a physician will present all options for care in a way that fully informs. Because at present the typical patient-physician encounter lacks full disclosures about options and outcomes, it does not well support informed choices.

Reason 3: Today's Physicians Are Not Trained to Adequately Communicate Benefits and Harms of Treatments in Ways That Allow You to Know the Consequences You Face

A visit between a physician and a patient should be a caring, relationship-building experience. I assume every encounter between a physician and a patient is just that. But medical decision making goes beyond the caring partnership between a patient and physician. Caring for and having a wonderful relationship with a physician does not guarantee that you will get the best medical decision for your particular circumstance. This distinction between caring and informing adequately is an important one. Medical decision making and the communication required to inform you should be done, for sure, in a caring manner. However, it is equally important that what is being communicated informs you of the consequences of the choices you face. Too often, physicians present incorrect information or, at least, obscure information and do it in such a wonderful manner that you may uncritically accept poor advice.

Let's set up a *less*-than-ideal situation to illustrate how discussions may confuse, even if done by a caring physician:

PHYSICIAN: Mrs. A, you need a test. While I think the chance is low for cancer, we cannot leave a stone unturned, as finding cancer is important because early treatment really helps.

What does a "low" chance mean? What does "really help" mean? The videotapes of graduating physicians revealed another deficiency. Numbers were not used as part of the communication with a patient. The physicians used verbal descriptions for the size of the effects of tests and treatments, if they were used at all. Words like "rare," "uncommon," "probable," and "for sure" denoted size. Using verbal descriptions may be a reasonable form of communication if they correctly and uniformly denote size—how much—for all of us. But they don't; no information is reliably communicated with verbal descriptions, and no informed medical decision making can occur based on them.

A confirmation of the lack of numeric benefit and harm information being communicated is that patients, like the physicians in the videotapes, likewise describe their clinical situations in words. Physicians and their patients in tandem often convey information about side effects, for example, as "rare" or "uncommon." These nonnumeric and indistinct words are used to represent important numeric realities. These terms really have no value in medical decision making because they have no universal meaning. In other words, my concept of "uncommon" and your concept of "uncommon" do not share the same numeric values. (An example of this concept: when grilling, I use the term "rare" to mean that my steak is cooked thoroughly, but my wife uses the term "rare" to mean that the steak is barely seared. Using nonnumeric words like "rare" creates as much ambiguity in defining the likelihoods of a treatment's benefits or side effects as it does in culinary discussions.)

Try this experiment yourself: Write down the percent number that you would associate with the following terms: (1) rare, (2) uncommon, and (3) usual. By this I mean pick a number between 0 and 100 chances in 100 (that is, percentage) that you think reflects what each term means, in a numeric sense. Now imagine that I tell you, as part of a visit for deciding about prostate cancer treatment, that the chance of becoming impotent after surgery for prostate cancer was "rare." What do you think are your chances of impotence based on this verbal description? Some may say that "rare" means 1 chance in 100; perhaps to another it means 10 chances in 100. What number did you choose?

Researchers have noted that verbal descriptions of numeric concepts are confusing and hence do not provide tangible likelihoods of benefit or harm of one treatment compared with another.[2] When people were asked to assign a number to the word "rare," their responses varied by as much as 10 probability points (some stated, for example, 5 percent and others 15 percent). This is a "large" difference in estimates for a term that denotes a small number in the first place. To think about this sort of range in estimates of 10 probability points for a term like "rare," ask yourself if you would think differently about accepting a treatment if the chance of that treatment causing impotence was 5 percent or 15 percent. You may feel, perhaps, that a 5 percent risk may lead you to accept the treatment plan. After all, at a 5 percent chance of impotence, there is a 95 percent chance that you won't be impotent. What about the 15 percent chance? Now the chance is three times greater, perhaps too great for you to accept the treatment. If this is true—if a 5 percent risk would lead you to act one way and a 15 percent risk would lead you to act another way—the word "rare" does not convey meaningful decision-making information.

The term "rare" was, as expected, associated with the least variability in assigning numbers to verbal representations. The word "sometimes" evoked responses that varied by 70 probability points (some stated 5 percent and others 75 percent), "most likely" varied by 75 probability points, and "uncommonly" varied by 18 probability points. Thus, using verbal terms leads to patients misunderstanding the real risks involved, which is unacceptable in medical decision making. Yet, it is all too "common" for physicians to use words when numbers are required. Sometimes it is because they don't know the numbers. For one of my informed medical-decision-making patients, a physician used the term "large" to denote the effect of having surgery on the chance of not dying of cancer. When the patient asked for the meaning of "large," the physician said "a 50 percent reduction." The patient then asked, "A 50 percent reduction of what number?" The physician did not know. (In this case, "50 percent reduction" meant an absolute difference, between performing surgery and not, of 0.0006 percent, which is clinically insignificant.)

If you ask for numbers and do not settle for words, you will be on your way to becoming a better medical decision maker. Informed medical decision making is fundamentally an experience of numbers. New treatments are proposed and research is carried out for one purpose: to show that one test or treatment, compared with another test or treatment, lowers the likelihood of some adverse disease outcome. In other words, medical science does not determine that a treatment works; it aims to determine *how much* better one treatment is than another.

Reason 4: Physicians Are No Longer Trained as Well as They Should Be to Make Decisions with Individuals and Instead Often Decide for the Average of a Population

Malcolm Gladwell, a staff writer at the *New Yorker*, published a book titled *David and Goliath* that challenges our often strongly held opinions about what is a "disadvantage" and what is not.[3] His stories hint that our beliefs, for example, that small class sizes are always better, that more money is always better, and that going to a high-prestige school is always better, may be off-kilter at best or flat-out wrong at worst. His wonderful stories encourage us to think more about the truth behind our ideas and to remember that common intuition may be far from the truth while counterintuition can be correct.

I, like Mr. Gladwell, am asking you to challenge thoughts about who should be in charge of medical decision making. Common sense seems to say that physicians should choose. The counterintuition, the 180-degree turnaround, is that you should fully participate in your choice. Medical care systems, rather than individual patients, are presently the purveyors of choices. The system derives guidelines and "average" treatment plans that tend to force people who are ill through a homogeneous funnel of care. For example, if you have an elevated cholesterol level, the system directs, via guidelines and quality incentives, to lower the level. People who smoke are guided to a CAT ("computerized tomography, low dose," but CAT is used throughout the book as it is common vernacular) scan or chest-x-rays to detect cancer early. Men who are young and healthy are guided to screening tests for prostate cancer. These types of general guidelines suggest the same choice to all patients and fail as a model of choice for individuals.[4]

The present practice of medicine says that their guidelines give us an advantage. Yet, in doing so, the system may be grinding people to an averaged-out pulp. The goal of medical care is not the same tests and treatments for all. The 180-degree-reversed goal is that tests and treatments should be reserved for individuals who find them worthy enough to accept. It may sound counterintuitive, but the fact that differences have been noted among physicians in the numbers and types of treatments they promulgate to their patients means that physicians are deciding for the average of their patients rather than for each patient as an individual (more to follow). (Not by malfeasance but by fiat, in my optimistic view. Most physicians believe they are doing what is best. Decisions are meted out, unfortunately, however, via guideline rather than by the balance of harm and benefit from an individual's perspective.)

A cardiologist walked up to me after a talk I had just given on evidence-based treatments supported by the cardiology community. I described studies to the attendees in a "blind" fashion: I presented data about the outcomes for patients without identifying the treatment. I then asked them if they would use such a treatment, given its value. I was in essence segregating the data on actual outcomes from the physicians'

preconceived beliefs about the benefits of the treatments. The lecture pointed out that, perhaps, these treatments might offer little to an individual. I expected to be jeered; instead the audience was supportive. The cardiologist who walked up to me afterward, however, seemed upset. He told me that he felt awful about giving a patient with terminal cancer a medicine for her concurrent heart disease diagnosis. He told me he knew the medicine could not help. But, he said, "I have to meet guideline for using that drug with her heart disease diagnosis. If I stop the drug, my patient will fail guideline and my bonus incentive plan will be in jeopardy." He also noted, almost as an excuse of his actions, that nearly 20 percent of the patients at the cancer center were getting heart-healthy diets. If there was ever a "canary in the coal mine" story for the cross-incentives of physicians, their systems' measures of value, and individual patients' values for care, this may be it.

With this story as backdrop, let's examine more fully the problem of treating populations of individuals as averages. It is vital to understand that decision making based on averages deprives you of personal choice. If we believe that individuals should decide and that individuals will differ about how they value outcomes of care, then we should see different types and numbers of decisions made for patients with similar maladies, and these wildly variable decisions for similar maladies would give us hope that patients are really at the helm of medical care. Why is this? Let's set up another ideal clinical situation to examine this question:

- Three men with prostate cancer, nearly indistinguishable under the microscope, see a single physician. One man chooses surgery; one chooses radiation therapy; the third chooses no treatment.
- Three women with ductal carcinoma in situ (DCIS) of their breast, nearly indistinguishable under the microscope, see the same physician. One woman chooses to take a medicine and forgoes surgery, one chooses to have a mastectomy, and one chooses to have minimal surgery followed by radiation.

What makes these situations ideal? The three people with prostate cancer and the three people with DCIS obviously feel differently about the distinctive amounts of benefit and harm associated with the treatments proposed to them. There are two sources of variability for these patients: (1) the absolute numbers (and percentages) of people with outcomes of benefit and harm afforded by each treatment may differ based on clinical and personal characteristics, and (2) how people feel about the outcomes

of benefit and harm may vary. Since all feel differently in this hypothetical situation about the values of the treatments to them, they pick differently. Each treatment, then, was best for them. This is ideal. At the patient level, variable decisions for a single malady is a good thing to see.

What would this ideal situation look like from the viewpoint of this physician's practice? We would note, if we peered at all the patients with these diseases, a distribution of treatment decisions (for example, some percentage of patients getting surgery, some percentage not). This is the ideal view of a medical practice: different decisions spread out over different people.

What would, instead, be less than ideal? Suppose the physician felt surgery was always best, or best "on average," and convincingly made the case to each patient. In other words, the physician is doing the deciding, by promotion and convincing or by offering only a single choice. For the physician's patients, we would see not variable decision patterns but uniform decisions for all three men and women—all would have had surgery. Hence, lack of variation in the decisions that require a patient's input is a sign that physicians or systems of care, not patients, are making choices. Wouldn't it be extreme to see all men get surgery if they felt differently about outcomes? Wouldn't it be extreme to see all women get a mastectomy if they felt differently about losing a breast?

Yes, it would be extreme to see uniform patterns of decisions within a physician's practice because the outcomes of these choices are varied in number and kind. Hence, if patients are involved, different types and numbers of choices will be evident for similar complaints, but if patients are not involved, limited numbers and types of choices will be made. (Of course, if the physician is not deciding but just providing a service, lack of variation for that physician is understandable; for example, surgeons will perform surgery, but family physicians will not. It is important to keep this concept clear: when outcomes differ in number and type based on the tests or treatments chosen, patients must choose.)

Here are two nonmedical examples to further illustrate this concept. First, suppose physicians were in charge of providing shoes to the public. If physicians took our personal characteristics and preferences into account, we would see different types of shoes on their patients: you like loafers; I like flip-flops. If, alternatively, physicians allocated shoes based on what they thought might be the best shoes for all, on average, then we would all be wearing the same types of shoes—imagine everyone sporting flip-flops.

On a less silly note, let's say two family reunions are going on across the street from each other: the Smith reunion and the Jones reunion. The elder Smith is the planner for her family's reunion, and she loves kickball. So, in the planning phase, Mrs. Smith sets up a kickball tournament. On the other side of the street, the elder Jones, planning for his family, happens to love playing horseshoes. In the planning phase for his reunion, he sets up the field on his side of the street with horseshoe pits. On the day of the reunion, what would we see if we looked back and forth across the street at the Smiths' and Joneses' reunion groups? On the Smith side of the street we would see everyone playing kickball, and none would be playing horseshoes. On the Jones side of the street, we would see horseshoes flying and none playing kickball. This is a huge difference between the two groups attending their respective reunions; there would be 100 percent variation in the games being played *between* the Smith and the Jones groups. Yet, we would see no difference in what each individual is playing at *each* reunion—0 percent variation.

What would we see, instead, if both reunion groups allowed all attendees to play any games they liked? On both sides of the street we would see different types of games being played—100 percent or large amounts of variation in the types of games at *each* reunion. But there would be 0 percent, or little variation, in the distributions of types of games *between* the reunions (assuming that the attendees like games roughly equally)—both reunions would be a cacophony of games. When individual choices are the norm, we see individuals doing different things but little difference between groups of individuals. In fact, any differences we note *between* large groups of people in their patterns of activity, whether games played at a reunion or treatments meted out, should alert us that there may be too much control over the choices offered.

Up to this point, my examples have been made up. How about examples from medical care? Let's take a look at different regions of the country and assess if decisions are equally distributed within groups (good for patients) or markedly different between groups (bad for patients). Consider the following:

- For women with early-stage breast cancer, lumpectomy (minimal surgery compared with full mastectomy) was noted to be used in nearly 50 percent of women who live in the Elyria, Ohio, hospital referral region, while in Cleveland it is only 23 percent, and in Columbus it is only 12 percent. Such a wide range in the percentages of women in large geographic areas getting similar treatments in those areas—from 12 percent to 50 percent—is not explained by differences in patients and their preferences. It would be hard to imagine that women who happen to live in Elyria, Ohio, by chance, like lumpectomy compared with women in Columbus, Ohio, who, by chance, like mastectomy.

- The rate of knee surgery in Fort Meyers, Florida, for patients of similar ages and infirmities, is three times higher than in Manhattan. It would be hard to imagine that people in Florida feel that much better about having surgery than do people in Manhattan.
- Over a ten-year period, reported in 2002–2003, surgeons in Fort Myers, Florida, performed over 7,000 more back operations and knee replacements than would have been done in Manhattan for patients with similar ages and functional abilities.
- The proportion of men having a prostate-specific antigen (PSA) test in 2010 varied from 4–20 percent in some states to 42–58 percent in other states. Southern states seem to order more PSA tests than western states.[5]

These examples, and others, probing the differences in patterns of decisions made by physicians by region of the country and by provider type raise concern about who is making choices. These examples might jolt you, and they should. It is difficult to imagine how these sorts of variations in patterns of care between groups of patients occur unless someone other than the patient is making the choice. It is hard to imagine that people who like having a PSA test done, and who are informed about PSA benefits and harms, tend to move to the southern states in order to be more likely to get the test ordered. It may be that golfers move to Florida to get their knees operated on rather than stay for care in New York, but it is unlikely that this fully explains the variations in care over large geographic areas, unless we could prove only golfers move to Florida. (My brother-in-law travels for his care to warm climates so that he can vacation at the same time. But, my brother-in-law travels only after a choice was made elsewhere.)

In summary, differences in patterns of decisions is a good thing when we note it between individual patients, and a not such a good thing when we note it between groups of individuals. The goal of ideal medical care is to maximize useful, individual, patient-informed differences in the types of medical tests and treatments chosen.

Reason 5: Financial Conflicts of Interest May Lead Physicians to Prescribe and Promote Options for Your Care That You Might Not Want

This reason and the next—financial and legal conflicts of interest—are touchy topics. I have many physician friends who help patients make medical decisions, and they are servants to their patients' care. But they are not the only physicians practicing. It troubles me to tell you that some physicians may not have your best interests at heart when recommending treatments or tests for your care, even if they think they do. Unfortunately, also, some of the physicians most likely to have conflicts are those who shape practice by being involved in decisions regarding guidelines for care (more to follow).

The problem posed by conflicts of interest is that options proposed by conflicted physicians may be limited to their preferred, or compensated for, tests and treatments. Conflict of interest occurs when an individual or an organization serves multiple masters, one of which might corrupt judgments about the value of services rendered to you. Conflict of interest is, unfortunately, prevalent in medical care. The Institute of Medicine (IOM) convened a committee to address conflicts of interest in medicine, and its report is worth reading.[6] The IOM report focuses on sources of financial incentives and on evidence that financial incentives influence care. When and if you read the report (a major portion of it can be read online), you may be surprised by how pervasive this problem is.

The IOM report points out that conflicts do not just occur when a physician serves a pharmaceutical company or other business interest; they may also occur in the day-to-day provisions of medical care. A hospital's care can be influenced by conflicts: hospitals have boards and must perform financially. Hospitals make money, for example, by discharging a patient before funds set aside for the patient's care has been completely used up—hospitals keep the leftovers. Might hospitals then develop procedures to make sure discharge from the hospital happens sooner rather than later? (I saw a flyer at an academic medical center offering residents free morning coffee for "discharge your patient sooner" rounds). Might early discharge be bad for some patients? And what thoughts are in the heads of some subspecialist physicians when they recommend a test or treatment that they perform for financial gain? (Remember the cardiologist's admission above that he prescribed treatments based on an incentive plan—physician practices are being gobbled up by hospitals and "accountable care organizations," expanding the opportunities for conflicts engendered by mixed-up, guideline-based incentives like the one faced by the candid cardiologist.)

There are many examples of the potential for conflict of interest when guidelines for care are developed,[7] but a full review of research on conflict of interest would fill a library, not just a book. An explicit example of the conflict of interest problem is given by a study in Germany reported in 2012.[8] The study evaluated "clinical practice guidelines" to see if the authors of those guidelines may have had financial conflicts of interest. (Clinical practice guidelines are produced by specialty societies and even our National Institutes of Health to guide physicians on the care of a specific clinical condition.) The researchers found that, for the 297 guidelines they could evaluate, 49 percent of their authors (680 of the 1,388 authors) had financial relationships with the treatments or tests that the guidelines addressed. In another study published in *JAMA* in 2002,[9] authors of clinical practice guidelines produced from 1991 to 1999 were asked if they had interactions with the pharmaceutical industry. Half of the authors responded; of these, 87 percent had some interaction with the pharmaceutical industry (58 percent received financial support to perform research, and 38 percent were employees or consultants of the companies). More damaging is that nearly 60 percent who responded had relationships with companies whose drugs were being considered in the guideline they authored. Oops—if guidelines are being used by physicians for making decisions, and if there is even a hint that the guideline may be tainted, we have a problem with medical care's standards for recommending tests and treatments to individual patients.

We might feel we can trust that no physician, especially ours, could be befuddled by a relationship with a pharmaceutical company, hospital, insurance company, financial reimbursement plan, or special interest group in such a way that he or she would lose sight of the potential for biased judgments. I have heard numerous times from those associated with conflicts of interest that "I am not influenced by the relationship." A leader of a research program (a conflicted physician) once told me that physicians involved with companies are the best in their respective fields, and one study that surveyed patients suggests they may feel the same.[10] The viewpoint of the leader of the research program and the surveyed patients cannot be proven, however. We have no information about the quality of physicians with versus without conflicted relationships—the belief they are better is merely opinion.

We also do not have robust information from research studies about how patients might feel about a physician's conflict of interest. In the survey study mentioned above,[11] researchers asked about 250 people their feelings about conflict of interest between physicians and pharmaceutical companies. They found patients, generally, unconcerned; 90 percent of patients had "little or no worry about financial ties that researchers or institutions might have with drug companies." But this group of patients may not have been the group to ask for an unbiased opinion: they all had already decided to enter cancer treatment trials before the survey. We might imagine they would be inclined to support the physicians treating them in the research setting. However, even in this potentially biased group of patients, a deeper look at the data reveals that some patients would worry. For example, 25 percent of patients may not have participated in their treatment if their physicians consulted with companies; 40 percent of patients wanted disclosure of the oversight of the researchers.

If physicians who have financial or other conflicts say they are not biased, then should we worry? It would be nice to believe that financial incentives, desires to advance a career, and prestige do not influence judgments, but there are just too many examples showing that, for some, untying personal gain from a patient's best interests can be easier said than done. For example, in the above study published in *JAMA*,[12] 7 percent of the guidelines authors who responded were candid enough (it was an anonymous survey) to say that their relationship with the industry influenced their recommendations. This revelation, at even 7 percent, is concerning. It leads us to question if our physician might be among the 7 percent, or like those in the 7 percent. But those claiming some culpability also said that nearly 20 percent of the other authors of the guidelines were influenced by conflicts of interest. This means they thought that nearly three times as many authors of guidelines were conflicted in their recommendations than reported. I guess this also means that they thought about three times as highly of their own judgments as the judgments of their peers.

While it is unclear if there is a certain dollar value of a person's involvement in a company or a "cause" that switches that person from no conflict to conflicted, some data from outside of medical care studies warn that a gradient might occur between received compensation and actions. In one example, votes against a bill to reduce sugar subsidies tracked with contributions from the sugar lobby: if $5,000 or more had been received, 100 percent voted against; if $1,000–$2,500 had been received, about 68 percent voted against; if they received nothing, about 20 percent voted against.[13]

The important point being made from the results of this survey is that judgments about the worth of medical tests or treatments proposed to you may be biased. You can't be sure that your physician will even know if the information about the tests or treatments has been sullied by conflict of interest. We want a trusting relationship with a physician who can help navigate our care through medical storms. These physicians exist in the majority, I believe, but they are a silent majority. The exaggerated vocal minority, unfortunately, may influence the way the silent majority thinks about what tests and treatments are useful. Physicians with conflicts should not speak for how patients should be cared for. While none of us can know another's motives, even a hint of impropriety damages a professional approach to caring for patients. No one can serve two masters, and even a penny of conflict, in my view, is too much.

Even academic institutions have conflicts of interest. I know of academic institutions where nearly every leader of a subspecialty section has financial ties to industry. These academic places train physicians and should be held to the highest, not lowest, standards. I "Googled" five academic institutions, as examples; each has an office of compliance and keeps a list of physician/research faculty, all of whom must disclose conflicts of interest. Conflicts of interest statements from faculty were ubiquitous. I will not name the institutions I queried, as I know academic medical centers too well, but you can ask for documents from your hospital or medical system regarding conflict of interest, usually free of charge.

Concerns about conflicts of interests are noted in many blogs, magazines, and journals.[14] In addition, section 6002 of the 2010 Affordable Care Act states that "drug, device, biological, and medical supply manufacturers and group purchasing organizations must report financial relationships with providers annually. Manufacturers must report payments to physicians and teaching hospitals, and ownership or investment interests held by physicians or the immediate family members of physicians." Hence, patients will have access to a growing number of resources documenting that conflicts of interest have become too much the norm in medical care. In fact, the first information coming from the Center for Medicare and Medicaid Services database is staggering: in just five months of reporting in 2013, physicians in the United States alone received more than $3.5 billion in consulting fees, travel reimbursements, and gifts from pharmaceutical and medical-device companies.[15] If you and I want our best medical care, all conflict of interest must be eliminated.

Reason 6: Physicians May Offer Tests and Treatments to Protect Themselves from the Real or Perceived Chance of Being Sued Rather Than Based on Your Personal Preferences

There is another subversive source of conflict of interest that potentially thwarts your medical choices. It is mentioned little in the IOM report on conflict of interest described above, but it clearly exists and is perhaps more pervasive than financial conflicts: physicians using tests and treatments mainly, or solely, to avoid being sued.

Medical malpractice insurance funds are the coffers used to compensate for alleged negligent care by medical teams. Our malpractice system is supposed, also, to serve as a disincentive for future negligent care, a hopeful supposition. This book is not an exposé of the merits and harms for patients posed by the malpractice system. I have experienced the malpractice system only during an experiment; I was involved in a study of the effects of a patient safety expert (me) at malpractice mediations (attempts to adjudicate financial remuneration for people claiming they were harmed by care, before going to court). The goal of this experiment was to see if our hospital could use the malpractice system directly as a springboard for making patients safer: we asked for small amounts of monies from any award to a patient to be set aside for research to reduce the chance of similar events for other patients. (I was not directly involved with the process of adjudication and am not, certainly and thankfully, an expert on malpractice law.) Our experiment was a failure: we were unable to entice even $1 from anyone involved in mediation, despite pleas that the cases we were involved with exposed safety issues that could be improved.

Even though I have not directly been involved in malpractice, I am aware of the worry engendered by the potential of a malpractice claim. The fear of malpractice has led to what some have called a "malpractice crisis." One of the consequences of the malpractice crisis for physicians has been that they respond with "defensive medicine": when a physician alters behavior because of the perceived threat of malpractice danger. The altered behavior means that the physician may propose tests or treatments that are not intended solely for the patient's benefit but, instead, for their own. Defensive medicine, then, is a barrier to personalized, individualized medical decision making. Like any conflict of interest, in which a judgment for you may be altered by gain to them, malpractice liability concerns may alter judgments for the gain of "not getting sued."

In my mind, malpractice concerns are just another source of conflict of interest since your best care may be subjugated to another's gain.

Is the threat to your personalized choices posed by malpractice concerns real or perceived? Unfortunately, it is real. Physicians admit they alter their behaviors due to concerns about malpractice liability. In a study published in the journal *Health Affairs* in 2010,[16] 5–29 percent of physicians cited malpractice concerns as the primary reason for choosing one or more clinical actions when they were presented clinical scenarios asking for testing and treatment decisions. Another study published in *JAMA* in 2005[17] reported results of a survey to physicians in high-risk malpractice specialties: obstetrics/gynecology, emergency medicine, general surgery, orthopedic surgery, neurosurgery, and radiology; 65 percent of 824 queried physicians responded to the survey, and of these, 92 percent reported ordering tests, performing diagnostic procedures, or referring patients for consultation in response to liability concerns at least once. (This does not mean they do these things 92 percent of the time; it means that 92 percent had practiced defensively in these ways at least one time.)

It is not easy to document how defensive medicine contributes to the numbers and patterns of tests and treatments proposed to patients. As I noted with financial conflicts, it is hard to know the mind of another. But, it is troubling that physicians admit they alter plans in response to malpractice concerns. We cannot have fully useful, transparent medical care for individuals when these uncooperative incentives continue to exist.

4

Personal Barriers to Becoming Your
Own Medical Decision Maker

To this point, I have aimed my comments about potential barriers to your best-individualized care at those who may be caring for you. In summary, the inability of physicians to share in the outcomes of your choice, their lack of training in decision-making science, their overemphasis on population decision making rather than individuals making choices, and potential conflicts of interest (financial and legal) limit your personal medical gains.

In addition, you as a patient may harbor barriers that keep you from your best care. These internalized barriers include how you feel about time (both for information and for emotional considerations), how you cope with options for care, how you may regret the choices you make, and optimism about how tests or treatments may "cure" you. I have watched my patients wrestle with these barriers when making choices, and I hope that by identifying them you will learn to limit their influence on your best medical choices. These personal barriers are discussed in this chapter.

Time to Inform
You need time to become an informed medical decision maker. I have spent hours with patients until they and I were comfortable that they knew the consequences of the choices they were contemplating. One patient took over an hour to stop crying before she could move on to making a choice. Making tough decisions is emotional (more on this later); it requires caring, and it requires the time to make sure the patient is completely informed.

A criticism of informed medical decision making is that the time needed is not presently available in a typical visit with a physician. There could be, on the surface, some support for this assertion. A Commonwealth Fund survey, for example, found that physicians say they are rushed to provide care and that they have less time for visits with patients and colleagues due to the pressures caused by measuring productivity by the number of patients seen.[1] Physicians claim that they do not have enough time for any one patient, because enforced visit times are brief. Sometimes physicians are asked to see patients every fifteen minutes or less in the name of "billing efficiency." Patients, echoing physicians' concerns, have taken note of these time constraints. Patients state that visits with their physicians are fleeting and often complain that their physicians are overtaxed.[2] A medical decision requires time, but the amount of time needed for informed medical decision making is not provided by, or reimbursed in, the current medical care environment.

The reason for the shrinking time available for an office visit with a physician may be the shrinking number of primary care physicians. The American College of Physicians has reported a decline in the number of medical school trainees going into general medical care.[3] In 2000, only 14 percent of graduates from medical schools chose to go into a primary care field. In 2005, this percentage declined to 8 percent. In another look at this problem in 2007, only 2 percent of residents training in internal medicine claimed they would pursue a primary practice.[4] This is a troubling decline, because primary care, I assert, is the place to become informed about testing and treatment options, not in the offices of specialists.

The brief time allotted for an office visit with a primary care physician has perhaps, in part, increased referrals to "specialists" to do the work of helping make medical decisions. However, specialist physicians may be the ones who perform the treatments they suggest to you, so specialists may be conditioned to recommend what they were trained to do. The specialist care situation presents an ingrained, hardwired conflict of interest (see chapter 3). When it comes to medical decision making, your physician should have nothing to gain from your decision.

Also, adding more time for decision making by adding up brief visits with *different* physicians may not be the answer to better care. Despite the growing number of specialists, these physicians, too, are becoming busy, and their time to communicate is inadequate. Patients tell me that their visits to specialists can be over in minutes and typically end with a recommendation for a course of action. Mrs. D. told me that the total time with the seven specialist physicians she saw was just over two hours, or about seventeen minutes per physician. Mrs. D.'s visit with me, in contrast, took over four hours in three sessions. One solution to constraints on time for medical decision making is to realize that a single visit does not provide enough time. Adding up multiple visits with the same physician may be needed. If it takes ten visits, so be it.

Time as Emotional Space

There is a second issue about "time" to consider. It is not about the time needed to gather information. That is a mechanical issue: it can take hours, days, even weeks or months to learn about, understand, and reflect on a medical choice. This second time issue is more difficult to deal with: patients rush to judgment.

Most people who come to see me for decision making are eager for a choice. They want the cancer gone "now," not later. They want the heart blockage fixed now, not later. They want the best medicine now, not later. It is as if a hot potato of judgment is burning their hands. I find that the drive to get treatment as soon as possible is a major barrier for patients fully understanding their choices and, subsequently, participating in their own care. This time pressure is largely unnecessary, you will learn, even though it is a concern to most patients. For some decisions urgency is required, but most medical decisions require, and can tolerate, a deliberate and thoughtful experience, and this takes time. There is no known clinical "line in the sand" for the time when a disease moves from treatable to not treatable.

The limited amount of time you and your physician share may contribute to your sense of urgency. It may seem, on one hand, that the short visit time allocated to medical care with a physician and the urge to move quickly to a decision are aligned to get treatments done sooner rather than later. I recently talked with a man who had been scheduled for surgery at a first visit with a physician after only fifteen minutes of discussion. The patient was, in fact, pleased—he felt that the physician was "jumping to it." His wife, however, slowed the process, and the patient ended up with me in an informed-decision session. He ultimately took four months to decide his care.

It is impossible to become informed about a complex decision in a brief amount of time. A partial solution to better medical care is to realize that most decisions are not urgent and that you can take your time. One of my patients visited nine times before she decided. For this person, that was the time it took. I know of no studies that have examined the "right" time to make a decision. Later in this book you will see how medical experiments are done and what makes one experiment useful and one not. Despite my experience in science and my knowledge of how to develop useful studies, I can't conceive of an experimental design that would establish such a clinically useful measurement of an "ideal time" to make a decision. The desire to make decisions quickly is fueled, then, by something other than knowing how chronic maladies progress—they progress slowly. Most patients with high cholesterol, diabetes, breast cancer, prostate cancer, lung cancer, HIV, or stable heart disease, as examples, need time to understand options and the trade-offs that exist for those options. Most medical conditions smolder; they do not flame.

To be sure, it is daunting to face a diagnosis of a potentially perilous disease and the prospect of taking time to make your own choices. Some people deal with difficult situations by facing them head-on, swiftly. Because of these human tendencies, it is important to remind yourself to slow down when making your medical decisions. The ability to fully participate in your care is hindered by making medical decisions too quickly.

Too Many Options

Patients often, but not universally, tell me that they wish there was only one thing to do for their clinical conditions. They comment that they are dismayed that every physician they see suggests a new test or treatment to think about. Some patients say they are overwhelmed; it is hard enough to face a choice about your future with a disease without additionally having to learn about options for care before making that choice. My brother-in-law recounted that he no longer likes eating at his former favorite sandwich shop. Why? There are now eight types of bread, which can be either toasted or not, plus six types of cheeses, and then lettuce, tomatoes, and on and on. He told me he sometimes wishes someone would just hand him a sandwich, no choice involved.

Medical decision making can seem like the sandwich shop: it may be easier to cope with one option, in some sense, than having to choose among many. Some patients prefer to keep it simple—they feel secure thinking, perhaps, that if there is only one option for care, it must be the best. Other patients, in contrast, feel embittered if they are not informed of alternatives. I find that patients, intellectually, want to know options, but when faced with choosing they are taxed by the fact that options exist. But having options is healthy—it means you have a choice.

Regretting Your Decision

There have been intriguing studies showing that people may judge the "correctness" of their choices by the outcomes that follow. By this I mean that if we choose one plan of action, but then have an undesirable outcome, we blame ourselves for making a bad decision and regret our choice.[5] People who change their minds about which treatment they choose have been noted to bear more regret than those who stick with their first choice. Researchers have found that people may make their decisions purposely intending to avoid regret after the decision.[6] To be sure, if only one option existed, then our anxiety (regret) would ease over having to choose among alternatives, and later we would not be stressed over judging whether we made a good or bad choice. We may think, "It is not my fault if I have a bad outcome if I did not make the choice." I understand this human feeling. However, if we want to participate fully in our medical choices, we must overcome the notion of self-imposed regret, by acknowledging that it may exist for us.

Stopping regret is easier said than done. There is a persuasive reason, though, why you should relinquish regret when facing a medical decision: no matter how choices are made, *by you or others*, the outcomes of the choice are probabilistic and beyond your control. All you control is the choice; you can't will your way to good outcomes. Medical choices require trade-offs between uncertainties. Regret may be part of the experience of choosing under conditions of uncertainty, but avoiding regret should not be the approach to making the choice. The important remedy for regret is to be fully informed of the consequences of your choice. It may be more regretful to choose, or have the choice made for you, if you do not know what may or may not be in your medical future.

Cure: Don't Think about It

Chapter 3 discussed how the words we use to denote numbers could lead us to wrong decisions, and that words are inadequate symbols for medical decision making. But one word that seems to cloud informed choice more than any other isn't a number at all—it's the word "cure."

"Cure" is an emotionally charged word. It is the most common reason patients give for wanting to be treated. A treatment that is described as "giving a chance of a cure" can be too appealing. But seeking a cure may cloud your best decision making if a cure is not attainable. And unfortunately, curing disease is not a reasonable outcome in the care of chronic diseases. Cancer, heart disease, and many other chronic conditions are not curable diseases. They may be controlled, and some treatments may reduce the chance of having these maladies be a consequence to your life, but cure is not possible.

Curing means there is no chance that a disease will return in any patient treated for that disease. Surely, some patients never experience a disease's return because another calamity intervenes, but this is not the definition of "cure." An individual with prostate cancer, for example, may die of an event unrelated to the cancer. In a study of screening tests for prostate cancer done in over 76,000 men, about 8,000 men died during the follow-up time of the study, but only 94 of them died of prostate cancer—the others avoided that end, perhaps, because something else happened first.[7] Consider this unfortunate example of one of my patients. He was found to have terminal cancer. No treatment was available that would extend life expectancy. After our visit, during which we talked about pain management and support services, he thanked me and left my office. On the way home he was tragically killed in a car accident—the cancer, despite its advanced stage, did not take his life.

The clout of the word "cure," and also the word "prevention," was shown in an experiment. Researchers asked people to make judgments about the value of two hypothetical medical treatments aimed to limit disability from a disease.[8] These treatments were described differently, however. Researchers told people that one treatment would "prevent" and the other treatment would "cure" the malady. People were told that the outcome of the choice would be the same under both conditions. Researchers then asked the participants to choose the treatment plan they would prefer. Respondents, given that the outcomes were the same, should have been indifferent to the words. However, they were not indifferent: thirty-seven percent of the participants said they would prefer the prevention option; 21 percent said that they would prefer the cure option. This means that words such as "prevention" and "cure" carry weighty psychological meanings and may variably influence our choices. The way to avoid this psychological peculiarity is to avoid these terms. Decision making about treatments for cancer or other chronic conditions should not discuss cure but, rather, which treatment plan has the greatest chance of keeping the malady at bay as long as possible. Ignoring the word "cure" may help you have more realistic goals for your medical decision making.

5

Medical Information

The following headlines caught my eye (all from the same online news website, no less):[1]

> "Daily Bread May Protect from Cardiovascular Disease"
> "People Who Eat Lots of Bread Are More Likely to Develop Kidney Cancer Compared to Those Who Eat Little Bread"
> "Adding Folate to Bread May Lower Depression Rates"

After reading these back-to-back-to-back headlines, I grabbed a slice of folate-laden bread and made a sandwich. I became depressed, still, because I reread the headlines and surmised that if I avoided depression and a heart attack, I might yet face kidney cancer.

Much of the medical information you read or hear about in media outlets is worthless. Information presented on television, radio, and billboards is often based on studies that are scientifically unsound, preliminary, or presented in ways that fool rather than enlighten (a good rule of thumb is to ignore medical information presented in advertisements). In addition to learning how to use information from studies for your medical decisions, it behooves you to be savvy about what makes medical information worthwhile. To be an informed decision maker you must grapple with numbers of the added chance of benefit versus the added chance of harm when comparing options for your care. And the numbers must come from studies that best estimate the likely true relationships between tests or treatments and your outcomes.

There are two general categories of research studies:

- Studies can be planned to determine the *independent contribution* of one test or treatment versus another to your best medical care. These studies are called *cause-effect studies*. "Cause-effect" means that a test or treatment (the cause) is directly linked to the likelihood of an outcome (the effect). Cause-effect studies are the best to use for your medical decision making.

- Studies can be planned to find hypotheses, or hunches, that one test or treatment *may* be better for you. These studies are called *observational* or *association studies*. Making decisions with information from observational studies is risky. You will see examples that support this claim in following chapters.

You are about to learn how to judge the value of medical information. Knowing how medical outcomes are measured (quantified) and compared will help you discern what information to use when you must decide. I don't expect you to become a researcher or a scientist, but you will need a working knowledge of what makes some information useful and some not.

The glossary that follows introduces this exploration of what makes information useful.

Glossary of Medical Information Terms

Association. When a study reveals an association, this means that the relationship between the test or treatment and the outcome event is estimated only and cannot be proven to independently contribute to your care (compare with "cause-effect" below). Observational studies, not experiments, are most often used to look for associations.

Benefit. Benefit is the absolute difference between options in the percentage of people suffering an outcome directly related to *disease* (compare with "harm" below). For example, if 10 percent of people die with treatment A, and 0 percent die with treatment B, the benefit of B is a 10 percent greater absolute chance of not dying (or a 10 percent lower absolute chance of dying—the difference is the same amount no matter how it is worded).

Cause-effect. A study that evaluates cause-effect relationships between a test or treatment and an outcome more likely determines whether the test or treatment will *independently* improve your care over other actions (compare with "association" above). Randomized controlled trials (RCTs) are experiments used to determine independent effects of different tests and treatments.

Evidence-based medicine. This term denotes the study of clinical outcomes and their determinants. Evidence-based medicine supplies the numbers for medical decision making.

Harm. Harm is the absolute difference between options in the percentage of people suffering an outcome directly related to the *test or treatment* (compare with "benefit" above). For example, if 10 percent of people using treatment A have a side effect, and 20 percent using treatment B have that side effect, the harm of B is, absolutely, a 10 percent greater chance of that side effect compared with treatment A.

Outcome. An outcome is a clinical event. Outcomes are the unit of measurement in medical decision making. Some common outcomes are death, disease, disability, discomfort, or dissatisfaction, and specific events related to specific diseases, or tests or treatments (e.g., bleeding, pain, nausea).

Trade-off. A test or treatment option that reduces the chance of adverse outcomes caused by disease ("benefit") most often, simultaneously, increases the chance of different adverse outcomes caused by the test or treatment ("harm"). Hence, a patient must balance (trade-off) benefit versus harm when making a medical decision.

Truth-based medicine. This is my term. Evidence-based-medicine may supply the numbers of science, but patients must decide for themselves what the numbers mean for them personally. The patient's choice, informed by evidence, is the proper, true goal of medical care.

6

Understanding Medical Information from Experiments

The scope and reach of the medical literature are vast. There are nearly 20,000 biomedical journals. There are more than 22 million articles just in the National Library of Medicine's MEDLINE database, yet this database of medical information includes articles from only about 6,000 of the approximate 20,000 journals. We can expand our pool of medical information sources, if we want, by going to Google, Google Scholar, and compiled online medical resources that are too numerous to count. The medical literature is so vast that information from medical papers overflows into our everyday lives. Sit in front of your television and before long you see information about a medical test or treatment and, in the process, are told how good it is for you (followed, occasionally, by a blazingly fast unclear listing of possible side effects).

The sheer mass of information makes it tough to imagine that anyone could take it all in—it's a mountain, not a molehill. My patients often ask, "How am I going to keep up with all the medical information about my condition? How do I know which of the studies in the morass of medical information are useful?" I tell them it is not as difficult as it may seem. It may come as a surprise, but most medical information is not fit for patient, or physician, consumption. I believe you can (and must) seek and demand medical information from reliable studies. As you learn the process for making a medical decision later in this book, you will become aware of the need for the best information. You will learn how to be more discerning. You will learn that, happily, the sources of information you should read are fewer than you think and, likewise, are accessible. At the end of the book I list some of the most reliable information sources for your medical decision making. However, finding the information is putting the cart before the horse. Before finding and using medical information to make a medical decision, you must know what sorts of studies provide the best information.

Measuring and counting are fundamental scientific skills. Clinical medical science is about measuring outcomes under controlled conditions (comparisons). It is as simple as that—science is a counting exercise. Counting, however, requires diligent, accurate methods of measurement. This involves several crucial concepts:

- Tests, treatments, and outcomes must be clearly defined and must be measurable.
- How the measurable events will be counted must be defined.
- The conditions under which the counts are taken must be understood.

Each of these steps is prone to error. Here's a brief overview, to whet the appetite. First, it may be difficult to define an outcome. For example, if death is the outcome, that event is readily measurable, but if the outcome instead is cause of death, counting accurately becomes less reliable—cause of death is not an exact measurement. Death certificates are used to "code" for the cause of a person's death, and they can be wrong. For example, a resident in training working with me completed a death certificate for one of my patients that said the patient died of a heart attack, not the cancer that really took the patient's life. (The cancer had infiltrated the patient's heart arteries, causing the heart attack—cancer caused the death, not the heart attack.) Error in classifying the cause would lead to an error in counting the causes of death. If an outcome is difficult to define, it is difficult to count accurately.

Next, even if we reliably define outcome events for a study, researchers can miscount. For example, the measuring instrument may be flawed or the person doing the measurements may make mistakes. Also, people in a study can refuse to be counted. And when, exactly, we take a measurement may influence its accuracy. I research ways to improve pain care, for example, and if a pain score is measured at a time when the treatment being used to reduce pain is not fully working, the effects of the treatments may be missed. Finally, the conditions, or study designs, we use to do our counting may lead us astray.

Yes, clinical science is simply a skill of counting accurately. It is an accounting of the numbers or percentages of events occurring for the options for care being compared. Measurement means there is an outcome that can be quantified, and that the quantity can be reproducibly determined. Measuring things about a human being requires critical thinking about what to measure and how to measure it. The fields of evidence-based-medicine, decision science, statistics, and economics all use tools of measurement. Each of these can help us understand how to make a medical decision. But they are just tools of the trade—instruments, rulers of measurement, but not the arbitrators of the quality of the measurement. It is more important to know how these tools can go wrong than to know how to use the tools.

In the next chapter I illustrate the tenets of science for medical decision making by posing a thought-provoking, chin-scratching question that has puzzled many a researcher. I describe how science might attempt to solve the question and highlight, along the way, threats to finding truth in medical studies. It is a perplexing question. If you understand what makes it perplexing, you will learn why so many questions in medical care are difficult to answer. Peeling away the nuanced layers of this question will ultimately show what studies are best to use when you face a tough medical decision.

7

Does an Apple a Day Keep the Doctor Away?

When I was a child, we had a scraggly apple orchard next to our farm home in Michigan. Red and Yellow Delicious apple trees shared their fruit with me and the many worms that feasted on their (before its time) "organic" juiciness—we didn't do anything to protect the apples from worms. I ate them daily (carefully and slowly). Now that I have established my credibility as an apple expert, let's attempt to answer the question: Does an apple a day keep the doctor away?

Hypothesis (or Hunch) Testing

An apple is an appealing metaphor for health. My mother used to tell me a variation on the familiar saying: an apple before bed keeps the doctor in the shed (farm humor). She was extolling me to eat healthy foods, and growing up with this saying resonating in my head gave me the impression that apples were special. And this proverb about apples and doctors is only one of many sayings involving apples, reinforcing the idea that apples are special: You are the apple of my eye. You are an apple-polisher. How about them apples? One bad apple spoils the whole bunch. On and on!

An important principle of science is that a research question must be worth studying. One of the prerequisites of science is that studies are based on hypotheses, or "hunches"—in this case that an apple a day may somehow be causally linked to keeping doctors away. (I saw a cartoon once that took the proverb literally, showing a patient in a hospital bed throwing apples at a physician trying to enter the room.) Sometimes it is just these sorts of belief systems, or hunches, that lead scientists to test whether the hunch is correct. Other times hypotheses are based on results of prior, or preliminary, research. If we are going to spend effort asking a question about our medical care, we are better off starting with a good hunch rather than a poor one. Medical science is "hunch testing"; hunches spur us to find out if some test or treatment helps more than others.

Potential Sources of Measurement Error in a Study

The first requirement of science is now established for our question of apples and physician visits: we have a hypothesis, or hunch, that eating apples may be beneficial. But what about measurement issues? Since science is about quantifying via measurement, what complex measuring errors may keep us from answering our question about the effect of apple eating on physician visits?

MEASURING THE TREATMENT: AN APPLE A DAY

The apple in this example is the treatment, or exposure; it is the item we are studying to see if eating them daily might lead to better health, revealed via fewer physician visits. The idea to study apple eating is no different, conceptually, that asking if surgery helps when we have cancer or heart disease, or if getting vaccinated against influenza fends off illness during the flu season. The questions are raised by informed hunches. The first thing to ask, then, about any study in medical care is whether the treatment and the outcome events are measurable in a way that allows for appropriate interpretation. Will everyone agree on the definition of an apple? Is an apple an easy thing to measure? Is measuring the apple more like measuring whether someone died (with a clear yes/no answer), or more like measuring why they died (with shades of gray increasing the potential for errors in measurement)?

As it turns out, defining "apple" is more like the latter. There are many types of apples (Fuji, Pink Lady, Gala, and so on), with different sizes and shapes. They can be eaten entirely, including the seeds, or they can be peeled first, baked, fried, covered in caramel (my favorite), or mashed and cooked into applesauce. Hence, the treatment, "apple," is not a precise measure, and it will be hard to quantify. It may be that it does not matter, in terms of the effects on physician visits, what types of apples we eat, how large the servings, or how they are prepared, but we don't know for sure. If we are going to study our question the best way possible, we have to specifically define what we mean by "an apple."

This process of assessing the quality of measurement of treatments and outcome events occurs similarly in a scientific study. Editors are charged to determine if a study is worth publishing in their journal. They often start by assessing if the treatment and outcome are measurable. For example, I rejected a paper examining the effects of vitamins on health because it had problems with how vitamins were defined in the study. I could not tell how much or exactly what specific vitamins were involved in the study. I could not tell how much the researchers gave to patients or if the patients even took them. Hence, accuracy was not possible despite the fact that a study had been done. Are you getting the idea that studying whether eating an apple a day might be valuable for us will be a difficult scientific inquiry?

MEASURING THE OUTCOME EVENT:
KEEPING A DOCTOR AWAY
We noticed, already, that defining the apple is difficult. Second, then, we have to ask, "What does it mean to keep a doctor away"? Is our goal the same as the cartoon suggesting that the way to keep doctors away is by throwing apples at them? Do we mean that by eating apples daily we will never have to visit a physician for any reason? What, in fact, do we mean by a "visit"? Do we expect apples to stop us from routine visits to a physician? Most likely, we mean that we will more likely be well and less likely to have to go to a physician's office for an illness. The point here is that the outcome event—in this example a physician visit—is also poorly defined and would require serious thinking about how we might measure the visit rate in the first place.

The difficult measurement issues arising from this science metaphor arise in all studies. The lesson here is that the first question to ask when assessing how valuable a study may be for your medical decision making is how the treatment and outcomes are defined and measured. If they are not easy to define or measure, scientific quality is weakened—high-quality science is about specifics, not generalities.

MEASURING THE CONDITIONS THAT
MIGHT INFLUENCE THE STUDY RESULTS
The goal of research is to find out if a test or treatment is independently linked with better outcomes. The key word is "independently." What might happen if we do a study and find that a treatment is linked to improved or worse health when it is really not linked at all? How might this happen, even if we define the treatment and the outcome with precision?

It may have dawned on you that other confounding, or "tag-along" factors affect measurement besides defining the apple (treatment) and the visit to a physician (outcome). These issues arise when factors associated with eating an apple a day, other than simply eating an apple, influence how often people visit their physicians. If other factors are connected to both apple eating *and* visits to a physician, we may falsely claim the apple is independently related to doctor visits when in fact the cause may be another factor associated with the person who chooses to eat apples routinely. For example, people who are health conscious may like to go to physicians *and* also like to eat apples. If this is true, then the health consciousness of the person will be what matters, not the apple.

People may also vary in how and why they eat apples. Some may eat apples while they exercise. Some may eat the apple along with cheese trays; some may dip the apple in caramel, peanut butter, or yogurt. The important point is that these "tag-along" factors, and not the apples, may bring about the apparent relationship between eating apples and visiting a physician. Epidemiologists will call these tag-along factors "confounders." Confounders can make the hypothesized relationship we are testing between the outcome (doctor visits, in this case) and the treatment (apple eating) look helpful (or detrimental) when in reality there is no relationship at all. A great deal of training in research involves learning how to account and adjust for confounding factors. Some study types are better than others at balancing these tag-along factors. In observational studies confounding factors can play havoc, but even randomized controlled trials (RCTs) are not immune.

Let's examine a study that illustrates how confounding factors can change the association between an exposure—in this example, coffee drinking—and an outcome like cancer. Numerous studies have tried to assess the association between coffee consumption and multiple types of cancers. Some observers suggested coffee drinking may cause cancer while others suggested that coffee drinking may be protective based on contrasting case reports and case series (these terms are defined below) of patients with cancer. It seemed, by observation, most alarmingly, that those who developed cancer drank a lot of coffee. Along with these clinical observations, basic (test-tube) research suggested that some coffee by-products might promote cancer. Based on this background information, studying the hunch that coffee drinking may cause cancer is justified.

As one example of the many studies that have addressed this question, researchers tested this question using data from a group of people followed over many years.[1] One of the measures taken in this population at the beginning of the study was the amount of coffee the people drank daily, measured as the number of cups per day. The researchers then coupled this initial measurement with a later measurement from clinical data sources that included whether these people were diagnosed with cancer. Then, having combined these data sets, they looked for a link between the number of daily cups of coffee consumed and cancer.

And they found a link: drinking more coffee was associated with a greater risk of being diagnosed with cancer. In fact, increasing from drinking one cup per day to six cups per day raised the chance of cancer nearly 30 percent (which could actually be a small amount—we will soon learn how to understand the numbers used in medical studies). The researchers even noted that there was a somewhat linear "dose-response." This means that they found that for every two-cup increase in daily coffee consumption, the risk of cancer rose, directly and proportionately. Dose-response is a criteria used by some to suggest a causal link between an exposure or treatment and an outcome event. It seems to make sense: the more of a harmful activity we perform, the more risk we might naturally bear.

But, as I hinted above, sometimes intuition is farther from the truth than counterintuition. However, despite my tendency to like counterintuition, when I see the risk of cancer rising along with a rise in the amount of coffee consumption, I am concerned—these are scary words, and scary associations, and strong supporting background information suggests the link between coffee and cancer may be true. (I am a four-cup-per-day coffee drinker and would drink more if coffee brewers would lower their prices.)

But as it turns out, the worry is unfounded. We will soon find that coffee consumption has nothing to do with cancer—the hunch is wrong. How would we debunk the research? We start by going through the checklist above: first, examine potential ways our measures of coffee and cancer (treatment and outcome) could be wrong, and then consider confounders.

For the treatment/exposure (coffee) measure, there were indeed potential inaccuracies: people reported how much coffee they drank; researchers did not observe them, and, hence, their reporting ("self-report") could be wrong. (Items measured by self-report are precarious for research because they may be imprecise.) People were asked to report an "average" number of cups per day, not a range. And they were not asked if they drank their coffee at one sitting or if they sipped brew throughout the day, nor were they asked what they put in their coffee. In contrast, the outcome part of the measurement, diagnosis of cancer, is likely more accurate than the measure of coffee consumption, because the researchers could get this information from a patient's record.

The measurement problem with this study, most importantly, involved confounders: the researchers did not include other behaviors that might also lead to cancer and also be connected to coffee drinking. The diligent researchers, to their credit, did gather information about smoking habits. The study team found that there was a correlation between the amount of coffee consumed per day and the number of cigarettes smoked: more coffee, more smoking. When the researchers restudied their data with smoking status included, the linkage between coffee and cancer was gone. (Relieved, I celebrate the new study findings with a large coffee.)

The way confounders are accounted for in research studies is to subgroup people who have different levels of use of a potential tag-along factor and look to see whether each subgroup shows the same relationship between the main factor being studied (coffee consumption) and the outcome, regardless of the group's level of confounder. In the coffee example, the study population was divided by the amount of smoking: none to lots. Then researchers looked to see if the association between coffee consumption and cancer was similar for every level of smoking. In this example, the association with coffee and cancer was nearly the same at each level of smoking. Hence, smoking was the likely culprit, not coffee, as the risk of cancer was tracking up with more smoking and not more coffee consumption.

The best studies account for confounding factors, but these confounders are often difficult to pinpoint and measure and, hence impossible to eliminate. When a study fails to balance confounding factors well, the result of the study is not helpful. Observational studies, due to their problems with confounding factors, should not be used for your personalized medical decision making. If we happen to think that the association between some factor, such as apples or coffee in these examples, is true when it is not, and we act on the information by force-feeding apples or denying coffee, the consequences can be uncomfortable at best, calamitous at worst. Later in this chapter we will examine a situation that turned dangerous for people when physicians acted on the results of observational studies of estrogen. While some observational studies may find true, independent links between treatments and outcomes, the problem is that we do not have robust methods to assure us that a true factor has been found rather than a confounding factor.

Actively thinking about potential measurement errors will help you determine what studies may be useful. Questioning the precision of measures being evaluated by medical studies when these studies pertain to your care is a path to better medical decision making. There are bushels of problems with measurement when trying to study if eating an apple daily helps us. These same sorts of problems plague many sources of medical information.

Problems with the Conditions Used to
Count Outcome Events: Study Designs

Before discussing study designs, let's review the ways a measurement may be wrong:

- Problems measuring the treatment (such as type of apple)
- Problems measuring the outcome (such as visits to a doctor)
- Problems measuring confounders: other patient behaviors that may influence how the treatment and outcome relate to each other

Now, even if a study adequately addresses these problems of quantification, another scientific concern must be considered: what process, or *study design*, do we use to count tests and treatments, and outcomes. Since science and medical decision making are about comparing the numbers of people with outcomes for every test or treatment available for our maladies, science must count under accurate conditions; the better designed a study, the more useful the counts.

Five general study designs are used in clinical research to answer questions via counting. Of the five, only one is useful for your medical decision making. To support this claim, I will describe how each type of study design might explore the relationship between a treatment (apple) and an outcome (doctor visit) and point out how each may go wrong. Each study design is associated with specific threats to the soundness of the science behind the numbers obtained. Medical textbooks list study designs ordered by their presumed ability to tell the truth. But the first four study designs described below cannot most often tell the truth for sure and should be used only to develop the hunches for further study, not to develop information for decision making. Some researchers disagree, claiming that one of these four types, the observation study design, should be used for decision making, so I also provide examples of using information from observational studies that harmed rather than helped after better experiments showed the observational study to be wrong. Then, you can decide for yourself if you want treatments proposed to you if the only information about your care is from observational studies, rather than experimental studies.

THE FIVE STUDY DESIGNS

1. Case report: "It works for me."
2. Case series: "It worked for four out of five people asked" (or, "Four out of five doctors agree").
3. Case-control study: "It worked, because those visiting a physician were less likely to eat apples than those not at a doctor's office."
4. Observational study: "It seemed to work when we observed a group of patients, some of whom ate apples daily and some of whom did not eat apples daily."
5. Experimental study, or randomized controlled trial (RCT): "It did not work for those randomized to eating an apple daily compared with others who were not allowed to eat an apple a day."

CASE REPORT ("IT WORKS FOR ME")

What does it mean to you when someone—a single case report—says a medical treatment works? Suppose you have a headache. If you take an over-the-counter pain medicine and your headache gets better, this means that the medicine worked, right? Suppose you know someone who had surgery for cancer of the prostate fifteen years ago and that person never had the cancer return. Does this mean the surgery worked? Suppose you decided to have mammograms yearly starting at age forty to screen (detect early if present) for breast cancer, and on your fiftieth birthday you are cancer-free. Does this mean the mammogram worked to keep cancer away? Suppose your mom made you tea that contained small amounts of a substance known only to her that she said was "proven" to keep arthritis away, and at age fifty-four you do not have arthritis. The substance, what-ever it is, works, right? Suppose you have smoked for fifty years and never had a complication of any sort, and you are "healthy as a horse." Does this mean that smoking makes you healthy? Suppose someone says, "I eat apples every day, and I don't go to the doctor."

The statement about apple eating, like the other statements in the pre-vious paragraph, is an example of a case report, or anecdote. Case reports are statements of hunches, not of truth. Useful medical information for decisions cannot be gleaned from someone else's experience. Statements about any single person's experience cannot be used to determine if something is better or worse, because there is no way to make a comparison with another person who doesn't do that thing—without a comparison, no information about "better" or "worse" exists.

All of us recognize the power of stories. My mom's extolling of apples was appealing. I loved my mom and knew she would not knowingly lie to me. Hence, I ate lots of apples. But science is about testing if hunches are correct, not just making suppositions. We must dispel the belief that a single patient's or physician's experience is useful to you in determining if something is better for you or not. It is sad, but I still hear physicians say "in my experience"—when you hear this, be wary! Another example of this sort of medical decision-making fallacy is "in my hands"—a single physician cannot know if he or she is better than anyone else, because there are no comparison groups. Surgeons have been asked to estimate their rates of complications and often underestimate how many they have had. In other words, they really don't know if their hands are better than another's. I once worked with a surgeon who claimed to his patients that he never had a complication after surgery. However, he always sent patients home from the hospital in one day, or transferred their care to another team—he had no idea what happened after his patients went home. When I approached him about his overzealous description of his expertise, after a patient of mine recounted a similar discussion, he defended himself by saying he was "giving the patient confidence." Enough said—case reports are not fit for medical decision making.

CASE SERIES ("FOUR OUT OF FIVE DOCTORS AGREE")

What if four people tell you that they eat an apple a day and don't go to a doctor? What if forty, four hundred, four thousand tell you? What if four out of five doctors agree that an apple a day keeps patients away from them? A series of experiences is really not any better for providing information about a test or treatment plan than a single case report. This is because, again, there is no way to know if the apple is making a difference because there may be another four, forty, four hundred, or four thousand people out there who will tell you they don't eat an apple a day and they don't go to the doctor either. If a comparison does not exist, no medical information exists, no matter how many people say so.

One of the largest studies ever done was a case series not about apples but a poll about who would win the presidential election of 1936.[2]

The election was between Mr. Landon and Mr. Roosevelt. In this poll, readers of the *Literary Digest* were asked whom they would vote for; about 2.4 million of 10 million readers responded, and 56 percent said Mr. Landon and 44 percent said Mr. Roosevelt, a 12 percent difference. By any stretch of the imagination, this was a large study and a large difference in estimates favoring Mr. Landon. But when the election was over, Roosevelt had won by a landslide.

How could such a large study be so dramatically wrong? That poll was nothing more than a case series; the "cases" were readers of the *Literary Digest* who responded to the poll, and more of these said they'd vote for Landon. No comparison was made with potential voters who did not read the *Literary Digest* or those who did not respond to the poll. The lack of an adequate group of people for comparison led to incorrect estimates.

No matter how impressive the number of persons in a series of cases, no matter how respected the researchers, no matter how well meaning the people doing the reporting, case reports and case series are not sources of medical decision-making information. They may be fun stories to hear, but ignore them for your health's sake.

CASE-CONTROL STUDY

This type of study starts at the end of a question, not the beginning. With our apple study example, the case-control study starts with people who *do* go to a doctor's visit, not with people who *may* go to a doctor's visit. In other words, a case-control study starts with the outcome and looks back to see how many of those at the visit ate apples daily (a sort of "look-back" study). As an example, suppose a researcher goes to a physician's office and asks the first 100 people coming to the office, "Do you eat apples daily"? Let's say 10 say yes. We now have an estimate of the percentage of people who eat apples daily and also come to a visit. The clear deficiency, though, is that there is no comparison if just those who visit a physician are queried. The comparison group in a case-control study is called the "control" group. The researcher must find people for the control group who are not at a visit and ask the same question. The researcher may go out to the street next to the physician's office and ask 100 people walking by if they eat apples daily. Suppose 50 eat apples daily. If 50 percent not going to a doctor visit eat apples daily, and 10 percent at a doctor visit eat apples daily, then eating apples daily is one-fifth as likely in those who visit a physician. With this sort of information, we may surmise that apple eating may be connected to fewer visits, but we may be wrong.

Case-control studies may point to insights. In 1971, diethylstilbestrol (DES) use in women was linked to a specific type of cancer by a case-control study.[3] Clear-cell carcinoma was a rare cancer; only eight women were studied, and seven of eight had been exposed to DES before their birth. Nearly no one without cancer or with other types of cancers had been exposed to DES. The ratio of DES exposure in cancer patients with this specific tumor versus DES exposure in a control group was nearly infinite. This ratio hinted strongly that DES was unsafe. DES use in pregnant women stopped, and that specific cancer type was reduced. Another case-control study showed that smoking was related to cancer; again, because the percentage of people with cancer (cases) who smoked was many times (about forty times) greater than for those without cancer (controls). Thus, some advances in our knowledge about the putative harmful effects of some risk factors come from case-control studies, but only when the ratio between the case group and the control group is like those with DES and with smoking. Many results from case-control studies find small ratios, like 1:1.2. Such small ratios are unimportant to an individual decision maker.

There are many things can go wrong with a case-control study. In our apple example above, what if the researcher had gone to the street next to the physician's office building and, by chance, that street was across from a market selling apples? The control group (people walking down the street) and the case group (people at a physician's visit) would be so different in characteristics and intent that no useful comparison could be made.

OBSERVATIONAL STUDY

Observing outcome events in different people under different conditions is a common medical study design, but a problematic one, as noted above. The observational study is better than a case report or a case series because comparisons can be made. Observational studies are a form of a "natural" experiment: some people freely chose to take a treatment (apples in this case), and some freely choose not to. These differing actions by people create different groups, so a comparison can be made.

Observational studies are common and are likely to become more widespread in the future because, alas, better studies are harder to do. But you should be especially cautious should your physician use data from observational studies: they are subject to error due to confounding factors that are not, or cannot be, measured.

One of the most sobering examples of physicians and patients acting on the results of observational studies that were subsequently shown to be wrong was when researchers observed that women who used estrogens had a lower risk of heart disease, and the more estrogens they used, the lower the chance of heart disease. (Sounds a bit like the coffee example above, doesn't it?) In 1993 the Women's Health Initiative (WHI), a vast observational study costing over $600 million, showed among other things that women who took estrogen supplements seemed to do better than those who did not in terms of the risk of heart disease.[4] Several observational studies even before this large WHI study showed that the risk of heart disease was lower by 35–50 percent in women using estrogens. The effect was so considerable and so consistent in the observational studies that some thought it would be unethical to study the use of estrogens in a more rigorous, experimental, clinical trial. Based on the results of these observational studies and fueled by the consistent finding of a lower risk of heart disease, prescribing estrogens became popular, with the presumption that this widespread use would lead to lower rates of heart disease in women.

But the illusion of the observed benefit went away when estrogens were studied in such a way that the effects of the confounding factors were equalized in women who did and did not take estrogens. In the WHI, a well-designed, large randomized controlled trial (RCT; more below about this type of study) in 2,763 women showed that estrogen use did not reduce the risk of heart disease even a small amount.[5] A study published in *JAMA* in July 2002[6] provided even more damaging evidence contradicting the observational studies about the value of estrogens. In that study, over 16,000 women were randomized to take or not take a combined estrogen-progestin hormone therapy. During the study, the group getting the estrogen combination did not develop less or even the same amount of heart disease—they developed more. The use of estrogens in this study resulted in an increase in heart disease, stroke, and breast cancer. The effects were so clear that the study was actually stopped before planned completion, to avoid further harm.

Why the difference between the observational and RCT studies? In the observational studies, women with healthy behaviors—such as not smoking, participating in regular exercise, sleeping at least seven hours per night, having a pet, eating more fish, drinking a bit more wine, and eating low-calorie meals—were more likely to selectively use estrogens. All of these factors are confounders: each has been considered to contribute to health, but we are unsure if it is these factors per se, or if healthy people simply do these things more often. In fact, it was the healthy behaviors of some women in the WHI study that were linked to a lower risk of heart disease and better health, not estrogens. Unfortunately, these confounding factors often obscure truth about relationships between risk factors and health. People and their living circumstances are the most important characteristics for predicting outcomes of medical care and these personal characteristics are poorly measured in research studies, but they are most poorly measured in observational studies.

The treatment in the observational studies reviewed above was not apples but estrogens. However, you can now see how difficult it would be to study and know for sure if eating an apple a day really does keep the doctor away just by observing groups of people who do or do not eat apples daily. There are too many measurement problems and too many confounding issues to accurately separate the effects of the apple from those of the other behaviors. Those who eat apples daily are likely to be different than those who don't eat apples daily, just like those who used estrogens were different than those who did not.

Since observational research is the easiest (not easy, just easier than better studies) to do, and since more data will be available, for example, from electronic medical records, pharmacies, and insurers, observational studies may multiply. Many of these studies fall under the heading of "clinical effectiveness research," which is even encouraged by our government as a means of knowing (http://www.pcori.org).

Our brief exploration of these types of studies should raise your concern about the value of such studies for individuals making decisions. Just because we have lots of information does not mean we have the information that means a lot. The truth about whether our medical treatments do more good than harm is difficult to ascertain from case reports, case series, case-control studies, and observational studies. By becoming aware of how medical information is produced, and by accepting your responsibility and ability to participate fully in your own choices, you may nudge our researchers and leaders to develop better studies.

RANDOMIZED CONTROLLED TRIAL

In observational studies, the observed people act in different ways (some eat apples, some take estrogens, etc.), and we do not know the reasons that they choose to act differently. For example, which women seek a prescription for estrogen, and how might they be different from those who do not seek estrogens? Perhaps only a small percentage of the population can afford them. Perhaps physicians offer some women estrogens but not others, or some physicians offer them to all but others do not, for unknown reasons. It is difficult to study the independent contributions of medical therapies, or even popular ideas about what works and does not work for your medical care, when the people studied are free to choose from a shopping list of options, and their physicians are free to offer from the list at will. There has to be a better way to study the effects of medical interventions, a way that limits freedom of choice while simultaneously balancing confounding factors. And there is.

The study design that attempts to counter the weaknesses of observational studies is the randomized controlled trial (RCT). In this type of study, participants do not get to choose what they want: they are informed of the options at the beginning of the study and then are assigned by chance (randomized) to one option or the other, usually without them knowing which option they are assigned. RCTs reduce threats to best evidence posed by observational studies in two main ways:

- By *limiting* the options for care—participants in the study get either option A or option B, and they agree to use only the option they are assigned to.
- By *balancing* confounding factors between groups of patients being studied.

Let's return to our estrogen example and review the dissimilar results from the observational studies and RCTs. When researchers used the RCT study design, the independent value of estrogens to reduce heart disease was gone. In the RCT, the treatment was limited to estrogens, and the confounding factors were balanced. RCTs should be the backbone of informed medical decision-making data, despite their potential imperfections (see below). These imperfections are usually minor enough that you can use information from RCTs to make reasoned medical decisions. To make a medical decision, you have to be able to compare options and be reasonably certain that the comparison includes the best available information. The RCT is the best way to gather medical information for your medical decision making. There are some potential imperfections of an RCT you should be aware of, however.

POTENTIAL IMPERFECTIONS OF AN RCT
- Patients or physicians may learn what the test or treatment is, and that knowledge influences how well they participate to the end of the study—this is called failure to "blind" or "mask" the participants to the goals of the study. (The apple would be hard to

study in an RCT because it would be difficult to have people not know they are eating an apple. When people know the treatments, comparisons are harder to make accurately, and clever study designs are needed.)

- People who agree to be in an RCT may be different than those people who do not agree, making it difficult to determine how results from a group of patients in a study apply to your individual care if you are not like them personally or clinically.
- Different numbers of people getting one of the options in the study may opt out of the study, making comparisons inaccurate. For instance, some patients may have side effects of a drug that are not prominent with a placebo comparison. In this situation, people may nonrandomly and unequally remove themselves from the drug-treated group, while those on the placebo remain in the study. This unbalances the random allocation of patients.
- People may not take the prescribed treatment as they are instructed.
- People may take, or be given, other treatments besides the study treatment, thereby clouding the assessment of the treatment being studied.
- Just because we randomize patients to increase the odds of balancing confounders, it does not mean we will be successful— sometimes things happen against the odds.

The fun scientific metaphor of apple eating and doctor visits illustrates many of the problems scientists face when trying to uncover the best information. The more you know about the quality of the information about your options, the better you will be at participating in your care. In the next chapter, we practice skills required to take full advantage of information from RCTs when making a medical decision.

8

The Math of Medical Decision Making

In his book *Innumeracy*, John Allen Paulos points out how difficult it is for many of us to think of numbers touching our lives.[1] We are emotional, intuitive beings, and these human attributes are not measured by counting. Reducing our lives to a number seems demeaning when much of what is important to us is embraced, not ciphered.

Unfortunately, our emotional intuition does not extend to our intuition about numbers. In medical decision making, numbers count. Numbers would be unnecessary if we could perceive the sizes of harms and benefits. But are we good at estimating sizes and amounts in our intuitive, perceptive heads? No, we are not (well, anyway, I am not). One of my favorite college classes showed us pictures and then asked numerate questions about them. For example, we were shown a picture of Chicago and asked to estimate the number of streetlights, or miles of shoreline, or number of pizza shops; we were asked to estimate the number of words in a novel; we were asked to estimate how long in days, weeks, months, or years it would take to count 1 million seconds and then, in comparison, 1 billion seconds. (Some student would always blurt out "1 million seconds" in hopes of getting a laugh, which would jolt the professor to alert us to think intuitively in days, weeks, months, or years.) We were not given time to calculate the numbers—the goal was to train us to intuitively perceive the size of large- and small-likelihood events. Try it yourself: how long does it take to count 1 million seconds? 1 billion seconds? You have three seconds to answer.

It takes about eleven days to count 1 million seconds and over thirty years to count 1 billion seconds. (I wish our political leaders knew the difference during budget time.) My intuition's estimates missed by a magnitude of years. By the end of this class, my numeric intuition improved. I learned that size matters and that only numbers indicate size or amounts.

Try out your intuition—estimate, quickly, the following numbers:

A. The number of babies born per second
B. The number of babies born daily
C. The usual number of words in a book

Next, estimate the following percentages:

D. The percent chance of dying in a car accident over your lifetime
E. The percent chance of dying at home in your lifetime
F. The percent chance of dying in a day
G. The percent chance of getting shingles in the next four years without a vaccine

Finished? Here are the correct answers:

A. 4
B. 350,000
C. 100,000
D. 3 percent
E. 25 percent
F. 1/250,000 percent
G. 3 percent

If you are like me, your intuitive guesses were off a bit. These examples include large and small number estimates and different time frames. These were chosen on purpose to show how difficult it is to keep numbers straight in our minds without knowing them plainly. We are better at estimating at the extremes of the spectrum of large and small numbers, but we are generally poor intuitive mathematicians. In the chapters that follow you will learn a process for medical decision making. The process requires knowing the percent chances of outcomes associated with the alternative tests and treatments you face. The better you are at knowing numbers, the better medical decision maker you will be.

More about Numbers and What They Mean

While it is true that we have a limited ability to intuit size, medical science is not really supposed to be intuitive—science is a counting exercise. But science cannot know how you will feel about the numbers counted. Medical decision making is both a math and a humanistic endeavor: in science we count events to find differences, but medical decision making is not purely about numbers, despite the paramount importance of knowing them. With medical decision making, numbers are the starting point, not the end. You will see, in the examples that follow of patients making decisions, that numbers help them use the emotional aspects of their lives to fully participate in their individualized care. This is because it is in these measured differences where you learn how much better or worse something is for *you*. You cannot make a medical decision just with numbers, but you cannot make a medical decision without them, either. Comparing numbers allows you to grapple with the emotional trade-off made obvious by the numbers. The numbers allow you to combine science with your individual preferences.

So, to be your own medical decision maker, you must learn numbers. This should not be a difficult task—numbers are a daily part of our lives. For instance, I went to a store to buy a sweater. The sweater I liked had been marked down in price to $100 from a full price of $120, and—today only—it was an additional 25 percent off the sale price. The salesperson told me, however, that the sweater was going to be 40 percent off in two days. I decided to wait to buy the sweater. I am not much of a bargain hunter, but 40 percent off is better than 25 percent off, isn't it? What the sales person did not say, however, was that the starting price of the sweater would increase to the full price of $120 before taking 40 percent off. Given this, how much did I save by waiting? If I had bought the sweater the first day at the store, I would have paid $75 (the marked-down price of $100 minus the 25 percent today-only reduction). Two days later the sweater would be $120, but I would save 40 percent—I would pay only 60 percent of the full price: $120 times 60 percent is $72. So, I saved $3: I would have paid $75 had I bought the sweater the first day. Plus, though I paid $3 less by waiting, I had to come back to the store, taking time and expense, and I took the chance that the sweater may have been gone (the trade-offs for waiting). Was the $3 saved worth the time, cost, and chance? That's the type of decision making we're talking about.

If you can appreciate this sweater-buying scenario and work through the numbers, you know much of the math of medical decision making. The example shares similarity with your medical choices and requires a balancing act of potential gain versus potential loss. Here are some mathematical truths raised by this example:

- Relative numbers mean little; 25 percent versus 40 percent seems a large difference, but these are relative numbers that have meaning only in terms of the starting cost.
- Given that relative numbers do not tell the truth about the actual differences, only absolute differences matter.
- There is always a trade-off between benefit (in this case saving more) and harm (in this case, time and expense to return to the store, and the risk of losing out on the sweater).

The following examples let you practice the math skills you need to make your own medical choices. These practice examples include calculating percentages, subtracting percentages, and building ratios. These examples illustrate how harm and benefit, despite being different outcomes of care (one related to the disease, the other related to the treatment) are managed with the same skills.

Math Examples

Example 1. The virus that causes chicken pox never leaves our body once we become infected. The virus nests in nerve tissue and can reappear years after an original infection. The reappearance occurs in the form of shingles, which can be painful; avoiding shingles would be helpful. There is a vaccine for shingles; it reduces your chance of having shingles if you are over sixty years of age from about 3 percent to 1.5 percent. What is the difference in the percent chance of shingles should you take the vaccine rather than not?

The answer is 1.5 percent: 3 percent without the vaccine minus 1.5 percent with the vaccine is a difference of 1.5 percent.

Example 2. If 10 out of 100 people who eat apples go to a doctor and 20 out of 100 people who don't eat apples go to a doctor, what is the added number of people out of 100 who don't eat apples and who go to a doctor?

The answer is 10 out of 100: 20 of 100 who don't eat apples minus 10 of 100 who do eat apples is 10 people. This number is calculated by simply subtracting the number of people out of 100 people who go to the physician for both apple-eating and non-apple-eating groups. Again, subtraction is *the* most important decision-making math skill. (I could make it more complicated, but my aim is to convince, not confuse.) If you can subtract two numbers, you can recognize how much better or worse one treatment is than another.

Example 3. If 10 out of 50 people who eat apples go to a doctor, and if 20 out of 100 people who don't eat apples go to a doctor, how many *more* people per 100 who don't eat apples go to a doctor?

The answer is 0 out of 100, or 0 percent. This is because the same percentages of people (number per 100 people) go to doctors in both groups (apple eaters and noneaters): 20/100 is 20 percent, and 10/50 is 20 percent. This example shows that it is imperative that outcomes be measured in percentages. In this example, there were, again, 10 more people visiting a physician in the non-apple-eating group (20 in the not eating group minus 10 in the eating group), but the number of people studied was 100 in that group, compared to only 50 in the apple-eating group. Outcomes must be "standardized" by converting counts into a percentage (number of events out of 100 possible events). While it is helpful to know how many actual people are affected differently when comparing treatments, that number must be also converted to a percentage so you can make meaningful comparisons. A percentage, then, is the number of people having an outcome event, divided by the total number of people in the study getting the specified treatment.

Percentages, rather than probabilities, are easiest to understand because we are bombarded with percent chances of things occurring. For example, my first look at my phone in the morning is at the weather app, which shows me the percent chance of rain or snow in my area (area is the unit of measure for weather). That application tells me there is a 30 percent chance of snow somewhere in my area (and it is April, for goodness sake!).

Example 4. Suppose you go to a store to buy a bag of sugar (a must for coffee). At store A, a bag of sugar costs $2.50. At store B it costs $3. How much more, absolutely, does the bag of sugar cost at store B than at store A?

The answer, of course, is 50 cents. (If sugar is sugar, the $2.50 brand is a better deal.) I include this example to show that if you can subtract, you can make medical decisions.

Example 5. Suppose the bag of sugar at store A was $2 and the bag of sugar at store B was $4 dollars. Now the difference, absolutely, is $2. But, what is the relative difference? (Relative means what it says: one price compared in a relative manner to the other price.)

The answer: Since store A's bag of sugar was $2 and store B's was $4, store A's sugar is one-half as much as store B's sugar ($2/$4). This is a 50 percent reduction in price ($2 divided by $4, then multiplied by 100 = 50 percent). On the other hand, store B's bag of sugar costs twice the cost of store A's bag of sugar. This is a 100 percent increase in price at store B: $2 dollars more divided by the $2 price of the lesser-cost sugar is $2/$2, or 100 percent greater price.

Notice in this example how big the relative numbers (50 percent and 100 percent) are compared with the absolute price difference of $2. Relative percentages are larger numbers than absolute numbers but relative numbers can fool us because their meaning depends on what absolute number it is relative to (that is, the number we started with). The difference between relative and absolute numbers is a crucial concept for decision making. Why? Because much of the time, purveyors of medical therapies make things sound better than they really are, and they often do so by using relative numbers for outcomes rather than absolute numbers when describing their products.

As an illustration, what does this statement mean to you: "Using this new drug for condition X will lower your risk of heart disease 30 percent." This sounds impressive. I sure would like my risk of heart disease to be 30 percent lower. But this 30 percent reduction could be either enormous or miniscule. What if *my* chance of having heart disease without taking the drug is 100 percent? After taking the drug, my chance of heart disease would drop 30 percent to a new percentage, for me, of 70 percent. This would be a substantial improvement. But what if my chance of heart disease without the drug is only 1 percent. How do I drop, absolutely, 30 percent from a starting percentage of 1 percent? I can't—a relative drop of 30 percent from a starting point of 1 percent would only be an absolute drop of 0.3 percent, not 30 percent. Maybe the 30 percent drop is not such a bargain after all.

Table 1 shows that the same *relative* drop in the chance of an outcome will mean different things to you, depending on your starting likelihood of the outcome event. Note that the *absolute* drop in column 3 varies based on the starting number in the first column. (The absolute amount is calculated by multiplying the percentages in the first two columns.)

Relative percentages, then, can misrepresent truth. I attended a lecture at an academic medical center by a physician who had a point to make about how patients with diabetes should be treated. (The physician

Table 1. Relative versus Absolute Numbers

STARTING PERCENT	RELATIVE DROP	ABSOLUTE DROP
100 percent	50 percent	50 percent
50 percent	50 percent	25 percent
10 percent	50 percent	5 percent
1 percent	50 percent	0.5 percent

had a conflict of interest; she was on the speaker's bureau [paid to give talks] for the pharmaceutical company that developed the treatment she was discussing, and the company prepared the materials used for the lecture.) During the talk, she presented the benefit percent differences in relative numbers and the harm percent differences in absolute numbers. This presentation, then, made the treatment look more helpful than it was (bigger numbers for benefit and smaller numbers for harm). The attendees' applause at the end of the presentation was misplaced—they had been fooled.

I tried to introduce a bill in Illinois to not allow relative numbers to be reported in television ads, newspapers, or any publication that would be read by the public. My concern was, and still is, that the use of relative percentages could lead people to misestimate the true values of medical treatments. I did not get far in my pursuit of this bill—lobbyists killed it. There is, unfortunately, too much at stake for some in the medical system to allow the public to know the absolute numbers of harm and benefit. But, there is even more at stake for you, as a medical decision maker, if you don't know absolute differences.

Example 6. Suppose treatment A is given to 100 people with pneumonia and it saves 93 out of 100 people. However, if treatment B is given to 100 with pneumonia rather than treatment A, 70 out of 100 people are saved. How many more people out of 100 people with pneumonia would be saved if treatment A were given rather than treatment B?

The answer is, again, just the subtracted difference in the percent saved: 93/100 in one, 70/100 in the other; the difference is 23 people out of 100, or 23 percent are additionally saved with treatment A.

Example 7. If 11 percent of people develop heart disease with a treatment, what percentage do not?

The answer is the reciprocal, 89 percent: 100 percent of the people being studied and who take the treatment minus 11 percent of people taking the treatment who develop heart disease is 89 percent.

This example seems, perhaps, humdrum—in a study comparing two treatments, an event occurs or does not occur in groups of patients being studied. But I have found that many patients get confused about numbers, especially when they are facing a medical decision. Even physicians get confused about the reciprocal of having an event occur versus not having an event occur. Some get so confused that they think *benefit* is defined as the reciprocal of having an adverse outcome caused by a disease, rather than the difference between one treatment and another. To be clearer: in this example, some might have said the benefit number is 89 percent, but that is not correct.

Benefit percentages may be communicated to you as a *reduced chance* that an adverse outcome *will* occur, or as an *increased chance* that the adverse outcome *will not* occur. The point is that no matter how you think about some event—as happening or as not happening—the difference number is the crucial number, and that difference number will be the same no matter how you think about the outcome event numbers. Some people prefer benefit communicated in terms of an increase in the chance of being well; some people prefer benefit communicated in terms of a reduction in the chance of not being well. It does not matter which way is used. For example, the difference between 11.5 percent and 11 percent will be the same difference as between 88.5 percent and 89 percent: both are a half percent increase in the chance of being well, *and* a half percent reduction in the chance of not being well.

Example 8. Now, let's consider another sugar story—not a bag of sugar in a store but sugar in your body. Blood sugar levels are kept in a narrow range by a marvelous, hardwired control system. It works like this: when I drink a cup of coffee with too much sugar, my blood sugar rises. My body notices this rise and sends out additional insulin to blunt it, thereby keeping my blood sugar level on an even keel. People with type 2 diabetes lose some of this built-in control system and must supply insulin via injection.

If the blood sugar value is high on a regular basis, the risk of adverse outcome events, like heart disease, rise. On the other hand, if the blood sugar value is too low, hypoglycemia (low blood sugar) ensues, which can be dangerous. Hence, patients monitor and adjust the dose of insulin to balance the chances of their blood sugar values being too high or too low. This sounds good in theory, but some physicians and patients use higher doses of insulin, aiming for a blood sugar value closer to normal, thereby risking hypoglycemia, while others use lower doses of insulin to let the blood sugar value rise to avoid hypoglycemia. Thus, there are two treatments: (1) higher doses of insulin to keep blood sugar levels near normal ("aggressive control") and (2) lower doses of insulin to allow blood sugar levels to climb above normal ("usual control").

Aggressive or usual control—which is "best" for a diabetic patient? To answer this question, of course, a diabetic patient must know the consequences of following one or the other of these plans. The decision presents a dilemma, a higher chance of being well (disease related = benefit) and higher chance of having hypoglycemia (treatment related = harm). This is the trade-off a person with diabetes might have to make. The task is to know how much better (benefit) and how much worse (harm) you might be if you choose aggressive control. How might all the needed information for this decision be shown to a patient?

Figure 1 introduces a common format for showing this type of information. It is the way I show data to patients and the one I use in this book. The figure includes lots of information:

- The number of people studied and important information about them, such as their average age (in the box at the top).
- The two treatment plans and the number of people in each plan (alongside the arrows).
- The outcomes measured in the study (the left-hand column— "Death," "Major event," and "Low blood sugar").
- The percentages of people having each outcome for each treatment plan (the two middle columns).
- The difference in the percentages for each outcome (the last column). This is the most important information for medical decision making: it depicts the benefit (major event) and harm (low blood sugar) of aggressive control. (Harm outcomes are italicized in all figures.)
- A balance graph visually depicting the trade-off of the harm versus the benefit (to the right of the table).
- The "trade-off"—the harm:benefit ratio (under the graph; more on this later).

("Major event" needs some explanation. It is a summary measure of numerous types of outcomes, such as having a heart attack, being admitted to a hospital, or having a stroke. It is a complex outcome measure because it includes some apples and some oranges. For now, consider it a single, serious *adverse* outcome related to having diabetes).

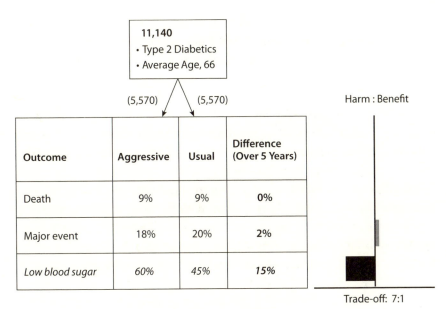

Outcome	Aggressive	Usual	Difference (Over 5 Years)
Death	9%	9%	0%
Major event	18%	20%	2%
Low blood sugar	*60%*	*45%*	*15%*

Trade-off: 7:1

Figure 1. Aggressive versus Usual Care for Type 2 Diabetes

To fully understand the numbers, let's first go through each row of the table in figure 1, starting with the row labeled "Death."

- In this study, 9 percent died in five years no matter which plan was followed (row 1). The difference, of course, is 0 percent. Hence, based on this outcome alone, the choice between aggressive and usual control is a toss-up.
- However, the percentage of people having a major event in five years differs (row 2): 18 percent with aggressive control and 20 percent with usual control. The difference is 2 percent over five years (20 percent – 18 percent = 2 percent). Hence, based on this outcome alone, aggressive control reduces the chance of a major event in five years by 2 percent.
- But there is a trade-off: low blood sugar (row 3) occurs in 15 percent more patients over five years if aggressive control is chosen (60 percent – 45 percent = 15 percent).
- The difference numbers, again, are the *added* chance of better outcomes (benefit) and *added* chance of worse outcomes (harm).
- In summary, with aggressive control 15 percent more patients experience harm, but 2 percent more patients benefit compared with usual treatment.

Figure 1 shows one of many ways to display information. I have used numerous formats with patients, but I have found that they learn most with this presentation. Patients like the figure because it summarizes information in a concise format. Some researchers use an alternative format called "icon arrays": a box containing 100 circles, depicting 100 people, with some circles colored to depict the number of people experiencing an outcome. In an icon array, for the diabetes example, fifteen extra people would be shown as harmed, and two extra people would be shown as not having a major event. The array is supposed to be an easy way to intuit percentages. But it takes many figures to show multiple outcomes, and putting all the outcome differences on a single array can be confusing, I have found, so I don't use them with patients. However, there should be no contest between ways to inform; any or all methods should be used if they help you. I often test patients who consult with me to make sure they know their numbers, and I will use any method I can to help.

Many studies have tested treatments for patients with diabetes. For example, a query in 2010–2011 using the terms "intensive," "insulin," and "type 2 diabetes" in the MEDLINE literature-searching database at the National Library of Medicine revealed 1,645 papers. Then filtering these papers to show only the ones connected with the term "randomized controlled trial" resulted in 306 papers. The study I described here[2] does not reflect all studies on the topic nor is it necessarily the best study on the topic—I merely use it to show how numbers are used in medical decision making, as the numbers in this study are readily understandable.

Example 9. In the above example of diabetes care, the difference in the percent chance of a major event in five years was 2 percent, and the difference in the percent chance of hypoglycemia in five years was 15 percent. What is the ratio of harm to benefit? What is the ratio of benefit to harm?

The ratio of harm to benefit (harm:benefit ratio) for aggressive control, then, is 7:1, or, there is seven times greater chance that additional harm might occur than additional benefit (15 percent is to 2 percent as 7 percent is to 1 percent, or 7:1). The ratio of benefit to harm (benefit:harm ratio) is the opposite, 1:7. It does not matter which way you look at the ratio—the relationship between the benefit and harm is the same. I use the harm:benefit ratio format because most presentations of ratios start with loss, or harm, versus win, or benefit. For example, the ratio for the Chicago Bulls to win the NBA championship in 2016 is 12:1. This means they have twelve times the odds not to win the championship as to win.

In figure 1, this trade-off ratio, 7:1, is shown in two ways: a balance graph helps you visualize the size of the difference, and the exact ratio is written below the balance graph. To decide between aggressive and usual control (or any decision you face), you will have to balance the differences in outcomes of harm and benefit for the choices available, so the trade-off ratio is emphasized in the graph. The balance graph is just one way to show differences visually.

The greatest potential amount of benefit or harm for compared options is 100 percent. For example, suppose that a disease kills everyone without treatment and that no one dies with treatment. This is 100 percent benefit added (nice, if true). And likewise, the largest potential amount of harm is also 100 percent, for instance, a flu vaccine that hurts the arm in 100 percent of people. Hence, the most harm and benefit you could see is 100 percent on both sides of the balance graph. The balance graph for the diabetes example is 15 percent greater added likelihood of harm (bar to the left) and 2 percent greater added likelihood of benefit (bar to the right).

Example 10. This example involves a three-part question about the diabetes example above:

1. How many people would have to choose aggressive rather than usual control to additionally benefit a single person?
2. How many people would have to choose aggressive rather than usual control to additionally harm a single person?
3. How many people will be additionally harmed by the time we additionally benefit a single person?

Making a comparison means that differences in outcome percentages are paramount. It is not that one treatment is better and one is worse; it is that one treatment is a bit better for one outcome and a bit worse for another outcome. This "margin," or difference, must be known to make an informed choice. I picked the words carefully in the questions above; I used the word "additionally." This word is a clue that you must determine differences so you can assess how many more people like you may be hurt or helped.

There are multiple ways to communicate this difference. One is simply to subtract percentages of outcomes to determine the absolute differences, as you have been doing in the above examples. This is the best way because it shows you the actual amount of harm or benefit you are deciding about. There are other ways, however, and I present them so you have heard of them. Also, you may have a preference for one way versus another. But you must be careful because some ways of communicating can cloud the actual numbers.

One of the other ways is "the number needed to benefit, or the number needed to harm." This way to discuss harms and benefits follows from the observation that a single person can't have 2 percent of a major event or have 15 percent of a hypoglycemia episode, for example. One individual can't have a fraction of any outcome—the only percentages that matter to a person are 100 percent and 0 percent: either an event happens or it doesn't. But percentages from a group can be used to determine the number of people who would need to be treated with one treatment rather than another before one additional (100 percent) person is benefited or harmed.

The number of people needing to be treated with one treatment versus another for either benefit or harm is found by adding up the percent differences until you get to a full, 100 percent person. For example, to calculate the number of people who would have to take the aggressive versus the usual control plan to benefit a single, additional person, divide 100 (the 100 percent person) by the 2 percentage point difference in treatments (100 percent ÷ 2 percent = 50 people). In other words, fifty people (each getting an average 2 percent added benefit) would have to use aggressive *instead of* usual control before one additional, 100 percent person might benefit. (Another way to state this is that forty-nine people would use aggressive control and not benefit.)

How about the harm side? Since the added chance of hypoglycemia with aggressive control is 15 percent, dividing 100 percent by 15 percent is 7 people (I am rounding to keep it simple). In other words, by the time seven people follow an aggressive control plan, one person additionally will suffer hypoglycemia while 6 will not.

The last question—how many people will be additionally harmed by the time we additionally benefit a single person—is a vital comparison. If it takes fifty people to choose aggressive control to benefit one person, how many more people are harmed along the way? Since every seven people using aggressive control have a hypoglycemic episode, the answer is seven: 50 ÷ 7 ≈ 7 (with rounding). Note that the number of additional people harmed by the time one additional person is benefited is the same as the harm:benefit ratio, 7:1. Hence, you can determine how many people will be additionally harmed before one person is additionally benefited just by the ratio of harm to benefit. I am unsure which way of presenting numbers of harm and benefit you might find most insightful. The only numbers needed for making decisions, though, are the absolute difference numbers.

Example 11. In the diabetes example, since the harm:benefit ratio is 7:1 (meaning that the chance of harm is seven times greater than the chance of benefit), should aggressive control be used in diabetes care?

If you were forced to make a choice based on a 7:1 harm:benefit ratio, the percent added chance of harm is greater than the percent added chance of benefit. Based on these percent differences alone (15 percent additional harm and 2 percent additional benefit), the choice is easy: don't choose an aggressive control plan. If medical decision making were based only on the numbers—percentages of harm and benefit—all we would have to do when deciding is avoid a treatment whose chance of harm is greater than the chance of benefit.

But making a decision based solely on percentages is too simple of a model to use for choosing—it does not allow for a patient's involvement in his or her own choices. Patients must weigh or balance differences in harm outcomes and benefit outcomes from their personal perspective. The outcome caused by the disease and avoided more often by the better treatment, and the outcome caused more often by that treatment are different outcomes in terms of their influence on your quality of life. One outcome in our diabetes example is a "major event," such as heart attack, hospital admission, or stroke, and the other is low blood sugar. You and I may feel differently about how these outcomes would affect us should they occur.

In fact, it is the numbers that inform us *just how much more* we would have to gain or lose should either outcome event occur, so that we can balance the trade-off and make the decision. How you feel about having to worry about and manage hypoglycemia versus how you feel about not having a major event in five years become the personal counterweights that give meaning to the differences in percentages.

Example 12. What would it take to *balance* the trade-off between a 2 percent lower chance of a major event in five years and a 15 percent greater chance of hypoglycemia?

I love to teeter-totter with my grandchildren, a love likely shared by many of us. By virtue of our shared experience, we know that we must supply some counterweight to balance the totter with our grandchild: the lighter child requires us to counter our weight to balance. The amount of countering force depends on the relative sizes of the people on both ends: the greater the imbalance in our weights, the more countering force we have to supply.

This analogy fits for medical decision making. For example, if you would gain more quality of life by avoiding a major event in five years than you would lose from monitoring yourself and thwarting an episode of hypoglycemia, then, your personal preferences may balance the 7:1 tradeoff. Your personal preference values for the outcomes are your counterweights to the differences in the percent chances of benefit and harm. Your preferences could, conceivably, move the balance to the aggressive control plan if you feel that avoiding a major event gains you more than you would lose from having hypoglycemia.

But how much counterbalance is needed? Notice, now, that the ratio of the differences in harm and benefit on this balance line tells you just how much more value you would have to gain by avoiding a major event relative to the loss from managing hypoglycemia before you might consider the aggressive control plan. In this case, since the added chance of harm is sevenfold greater than the added chance of benefit, avoiding a major event would have to be at least seven times greater gain in value *to you* compared to the value you would lose from being hypoglycemic.

Medical decision making, then, is a countering force, a teeter-totter balancing experience. The countering force is your feelings about the value you gain should you avoid an outcome caused by disease relative to the value you would lose should you be harmed by the treatment. And that determination depends on the person facing the decision. Two people, both facing the same choice, both presented the same percentages, may make different choices based on their personal values of gain and loss.

We are now at the defining moment of medical decision making—where science meets the individual. We are at the point where you realize how you can become involved in medical decisions, and where you realize you must be the one who makes medical decisions. Only you can trade off values of potential gain versus potential loss based on *how you feel* about differences in the percent chances of good and bad outcomes; no one else can do that for you. Informed decision making occurs when you balance how much personal value *may* be gained or lost when choosing one treatment rather than another. The ratio of harm to benefit sets the stage for you to know just how much greater or lesser your preferences for given outcomes will have to be in order to balance differences in outcome percentages.

But this trade-off of preferences for different outcomes of care is not an easy task. Decision scientists toil to find ways to measure preference values, also called quality-of-life values. There are several ways you can come to grips with the tough task of trading off outcomes based on personal values. In the next chapter I briefly outline the methods used by decision scientists, and then I introduce how I help patients make trade-offs.

9

How to Determine the Value of Potential Gains and Losses to Your Health

During my training in clinical decision making at Tufts New England Medical Center, I learned methods to numerically quantify a person's quality of life. The number assigned to an outcome of care would tell how much value in quality of life might be lost for having a given outcome. For example, we might try to determine how much value in quality of life might be lost for suffering hypoglycemia, a stroke, or chronic pain. Any outcome of disease or treatment can be queried for its potential to reduce a full quality of life. There are two main methods for determining the quantitative value of an outcome: the visual analog scale and the standard gamble.

Visual Analog Scale

The visual analog scale (VAS) sets boundaries for the best possible state of health and the worst: the worst state of health is assigned 0 points, and the best 100 points. All other states of health (outcomes) fall between these extremes. People are asked to put less than full quality of life outcomes on the scale between the extremes. For example, suppose you place a value of 80 on hypoglycemia. This means that you think you would lose 20 points out of 100 for having such an episode (or gain 20 points if you avoided that outcome). The values to gain and lose are always differences from a full, healthy life.

I confess, though, that I do not often use the VAS with patients. Researchers have noted that patients using this scale generally assign unreasonably low values for quality of life.[1]

Standard Gamble

The standard gamble (SG) is another tool used to assign a number to quality of life. The number obtained using this tool is nearly always different than the number obtained using the VAS. With the SG, a person is given a choice between two doors—a *Price Is Right* kind of choice. Behind door 1 is the certainty that you will live but you will also have the certainty of suffering a negative outcome, for example, hypoglycemia. Behind door 2 is a 50:50 chance of the best outcome, being well, and the worst outcome, death. After explaining the task, patients are asked to choose a door. If a person chooses the 50:50 door—the gamble—we know that avoiding the certain outcome is worth a 50 percent chance of dying. If this example were true, then the number obtained from the gamble's percentage is the quality-of-life value for the outcome event (50 in this hypothetical example). This would mean that you would lose 50 points out of 100 if you suffered the negative outcome behind door 1.

Patients never, in my experience, take a 50 percent chance of dying immediately to avoid anything (except maybe shopping, my son says). Hence, when conducting an SG session with a patient, I change the 50:50 starting percentage of the gamble systematically until the person is indifferent between the gamble and the certainty of the outcome. Typical numbers for gambles show that patients usually choose, at most, only a small risk of death behind door 2. This means that the quality-of-life numbers from the SG are closer to full quality (100 points) than numbers from VAS (this means you would lose less value if you used the SG number than if you used the VAS number). To give you a sense of comparison between the VAS and SG methods, I had a patient who assigned a number for having a stroke at 10 out of 100 using the VAS (losing 90 of 100 points should he have a stroke) and a value of 90 using the SG (losing 10 of 100 points should he have a stroke). Clearly, the value to gain for avoiding this outcome would vary dramatically depending on the scale used: 90 points with one and 10 with the other. Such dramatic differences in the values for quality of life are not uncommon when comparing these methods.

Like with the VAS, I do not often use the SG with patients. One of the first times I tried the SG method with a patient, the elderly lady scolded me, saying that she had never gambled in her life and she was not about to start. But this does not mean that you should not use the methods if they help you determine how much value there may be for you to lose or gain should you potentially experience outcomes for your disease and treatment plans.

The "Relative Trade-Off"

Researchers in health policy compare medical actions across populations and, hence, must numerically assign values to health states (another example of average-person decision making that does not help individuals). For an individual, however, it is uncertain that a numeric value must be assigned to competing outcomes for you to be able to balance harm and benefit. After twenty-five years of experience consulting with patients, I found that balancing gain and loss is best done in a relative sense. I came to this insight by trial and error. I suffered along with patients as they struggled to numerically balance one outcome against another. Patients would often, however, be able to balance harm and benefit outcomes even if they were reticent to supply a number.

I realized how to help patients think about the values to gain or lose after one of my patients, an engineer, told me that she could better decide about how she would value the outcomes of care if she could compare them, relatively, as a ratio. This woman was deciding about a treatment for breast cancer and had to trade off a small added increase in life expectancy for undergoing radiation therapy against the added chance of side effects to the breast and lung tissue caused by radiation. After I showed her the numbers for the added chance of benefit and added chance of harm, which had a harm:benefit ratio for her of about 50:1, she said to me, "Well, that means I better think that not dying of breast cancer in twenty years is fifty times better than having a lung problem. Well, I think it is." She did not assign a number to the outcomes of gain and loss. Instead, she intuitively made a trade-off by comparing the relative differences in harm and benefit. She felt the value to gain by the small, reduced chance of not dying was at least fifty times better than the quality of life she might lose should she suffer a side effect that would aggravate but not kill her.

This eye-opening experience taught me that people do not need to assign numbers to their outcomes in order to make their choices. All they have to do is consider how much more relative value there is to gain than to lose, or vice versa. So, despite my training in decision science, and after years of trying to help patients understand the VAS and SG, I started discussing with patients how to *relatively* value outcome events should they occur. I find this method helps patients make the trade-offs they face. So, when it comes to personal value evaluation, relativity matters. The harm:benefit ratios, for any decision, tell you how much relative, teeter-totter weight may be needed to balance the different outcomes reflected in the percentages. I have no proof this relative value thinking is best; please use any method you like to come to grips with the trade-offs you face.

There are books dedicated to the subject of assessing quality of life/value rankings. Some tools help you appreciate what the outcomes might be like should you experience them, breaking down outcomes into lists of symptoms you might encounter. Researchers have developed computer programs to assess if nausea or headache is preferred to weakness or fatigue, for example. In a study I did with people with hepatitis C,[2] I gave them a box containing a full list of potential symptoms that had been suffered by others with the disease. I asked them to check their own symptoms and then numerically value their personalized set. There are decision aids designed to classify outcomes for some disease conditions, such as the PANDAs model.[3] The best course, however, is to talk with your physician, learn the outcomes, and know the numbers you will need to make your best choice. Medical decision making is best accomplished with a conversation.

A summary of math skills follows. A quiz is included to reinforce what you have learned. The cases in the chapters that follow illustrate how patients used these skills to make their best choices.

SUMMARY OF MATH SKILLS

Science is a counting exercise. Medical science counts outcome events in groups of patients taking competing tests or treatments. The counts are presented as percentages of people having the outcome.

Subtracting percentages is *the* medical decision-making skill. It determines how much better or worse one test or treatment versus another may be for you.

Benefit: the numeric, absolute amount that one test or treatment compared with another adds to the percent chance that you will avoid some detrimental outcome that is directly related to the disease that you have.

Harm: the numeric, absolute amount that one treatment compared with another adds to the percent chance that you will suffer a detrimental outcome that is directly related to the test or treatment you chose.

Harm:benefit ratio: the difference in the amount of harm to the difference in the amount of benefit. The ratio allows you to determine how much you potentially may gain versus how much you potentially may lose in terms of your quality of life by the choice you are considering. The ratio of harm to benefit is your strategic starting place for medical decision making.

How Do I Present Numbers to Decision Makers?

Figure 1 above, for the diabetes example, is a graphical summary of information I use in medical decision making. The table and balance graph in the figure include information imperative for making informed choices.

Figure 2 depicts another study and, again, is presented in the graphical format used with patients in the following chapters. The study was done to see if doing a CAT scan rather than a chest x-ray (CXR) might find lung cancer earlier and thereby lead to fewer people dying of that disease.[4] The "Difference" column is empty, and so is the harm:benefit ratio and balance graph. Complete the table and balance graph. To complete the figure, you will have to determine the following:

A. The difference in dying of lung cancer over five years (row 1)
B. The difference in having a death or severe complication within sixty days after the test due to the work-up done for an abnormality on the test (row 2)
C. The difference in the percentage of people with a positive test but no cancer (row 3)

First, I give a brief description of the study, and the answers follow.

This example is a summary "quiz" before moving on to examples of patients making decisions in the next several chapters. I present it for several reasons. First, there are two harms: (a) suffering death or a severe complication during a work-up for a positive test within sixty days following the test, and (b) a false-positive test result (test falsely says cancer may be there). False-positive results are a bane of tests. A test that finds an abnormality will be unable to tell you what the abnormality is. Hence, more diagnostic work is needed to follow up on the test abnormality. Sometimes the abnormality is what we aimed to find (a true positive); other times it is incidental and not important to your care (a false positive; more on these in chapter 16). The CAT scan is like a binocular compared with the eyeglasses of a CXR. CAT scans thus find more abnormalities than CXRs, and some of these abnormalities are cancer, but some are not. The problem is that to discover that the abnormality is not cancer may require surgery (to the lung). That is dangerous, and more people died or suffered major complications shortly after the test from the work-up of abnormalities in the CAT group due to the greater number of people with positive findings. This example also allows me to present another way of knowing what numbers mean to you. In addition to knowing the percentages of outcomes and the numbers needed to benefit or harm one added

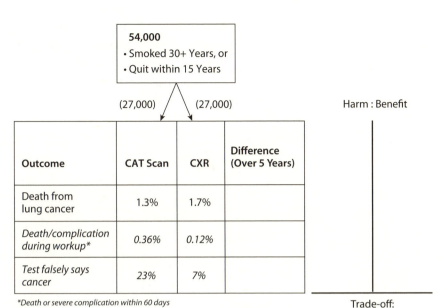

Outcome	CAT Scan	CXR	Difference (Over 5 Years)
Death from lung cancer	1.3%	1.7%	
Death/complication during workup*	0.36%	0.12%	
Test falsely says cancer	23%	7%	

54,000
• Smoked 30+ Years, or
• Quit within 15 Years

(27,000)   (27,000)

Harm : Benefit

Trade-off:

*Death or severe complication within 60 days

Figure 2. CAT Scan versus Chest X-ray to Screen for Lung Cancer

person, you can count the actual number of people affected differently in the two compared groups. For example, 356 people died in the CAT scan group and 443 in the CXR group for a difference of 87 people out of the 54,000 people in the study. However, not all died of lung cancer (the aim of the study was to reduce lung cancer deaths): 274 died of lung cancer in the CAT scan group, and 309 in the CXR group. The different number of people dying of lung cancer between the compared groups is then 36 (309 − 274 = 36) people out of 54,000 in the study.

Knowing the percentages, the ratios, and the actual numbers of people affected by tests or treatments will help you fully understand the consequences you may face. This example is a good one because small amounts of harm and benefit are not uncommon. It also shows why you must make choices: trade-offs between small difference numbers require your input.

Now for the answers for the questions above: the difference for row 1 is 0.4 percent, for row 2 is 0.24 percent, and for row 3 is 16 percent; the harm:benefit ratio for dying during work-up is about 1:2 (0.24 percent : 0.4 percent); and harm:benefit ratio for a false finding is 40:1 (16 percent : 0.4 percent).

You may want to consider what the harm:benefit ratios mean to you for this trade-off between CAT and CXR. This may take a moment to figure out. For example, the first harm:benefit ratio, death or suffering a complication during work-up within sixty days versus dying from lung cancer within five years, includes death for both outcomes. However, *when in time* death occurs is the trade-off for this harm. More people died or suffered a complication in the CAT scan group than in the CXR group within sixty days after the test from the surgery done to follow up an abnormal test finding.

10

Making Decisions

Two patients of mine, one fifty-five and the other sixty-five years of age, had the same problem. Mr. B. and Mr. C. both had prostate cancer limited to one side of the prostate gland, and under the microscope their tumors looked identical. *Both* were contemplating surgery. These men ultimately made different decisions, and in these different decisions we learn how individuals and their preferences matter. These men's stories are presented first; they are paired to underscore how different people may have different harms and benefits for the same disease process, and different preferences for their potential outcomes. Other stories follow: a man and his wife, also facing together a choice for prostate cancer treatment, stop their pursuit after learning that research studies have not addressed their ethnic group; a woman must decide about a medication, another about which test she should have to screen for breast cancer, and a third about whether to have both breasts removed after finding she has breast cancer; a woman and a man decide for aggressive treatments for cancer without any evidence of benefit; and a woman decides to forgo a vaccine for shingles suggested by her physician and is surprised by the physician's response.

In the following examples, I do not identify patients. As they say on television, the names and faces have been changed to protect the innocent. I have consulted with hundreds of people; the few stories I present were chosen because they are common decision-making circumstances, and they address common concerns that patients have when making an informed medical decision. You will not be able to pinpoint any patient; some gave me permission to discuss their case; others are gone from my care; yet others have died. However, due to their usual circumstances, you will recognize the medical decisions they had to face, and you may closely identify with them. The goal is to learn the process of medical decision making by watching these people make their decisions.

Each person presented has unique clinical characteristics. Do not assume that the numbers used for their decisions are the same numbers yours might be. I did attempt to present cases usual enough that you will learn about some of the best medical studies for the particular diseases, but one of the tenets of informed choice is that numbers differ for individuals. You may have unique characteristics that would exclude you from comparing yourself to these patients. The goal, again, is to learn the process.

Each case follows a similar format. This is a good time to revisit the decision-making checklist from chapter 2:

DECISION-MAKING CHECKLIST

1. Slow down: take time to decide. Don't let fear dictate your choice.
2. Slow down: take time to decide. Don't let fear dictate your choice. (repeated on purpose)
3. Know your diagnosis. Diseases differ even if they carry the same name.
4. Study the experiments that test options for your care. Determine, for all options, what number and percentage of people in the study had the outcomes—both good and bad.
   a. Determine the percentage of people who had the outcome caused by disease for each treatment.
   b. Subtract the percentages of people having the outcome caused by the disease for compared options. This difference is the added chance of benefit.
   c. Determine the percentage of people who had the outcome caused by treatment for compared options.
   d. Subtract the percentages of people having the outcome caused by the treatment for compared options. This difference is the added chance of harm.
5. Compare the difference in the added chances of benefit and harm; use graphics to help you understand.
6. Assess your unique clinical situation, and modify the numbers for your situation.

decision making is a personal process; you must decide based on your values for the benefits and harms of different options for care.

As for your second question about the time required, I'm not sure how long the visit will take. Some people come to grips with their choice quickly, but others need more time before they can choose. Usually the first visit takes about an hour. Most people, however, come back for more discussion. People often are only able to remember a limited amount of information at any one time. Also, making a decision can be an emotional task, and people get tired. Please let me know how you are doing as we go along, and we will be flexible with your time. Rest assured, however, we will take as much time as you need to be sure you are fully informed about your decision.

MR. B.: I am glad we will have time. I have been to three doctors about my cancer, and the total time with all three is less than one hour. I have been rushed around and haven't really had a chance to figure this thing out.

ME: Why don't you tell me what has been happening to you, step by step?

MR. B.: I went to see my primary doctor in February for a regular exam scheduled for executives at my company, and he ordered a blood test, which he said would screen for prostate cancer. The test came back with an elevated level, which I was told may or may not indicate cancer. The test was repeated and the result was still elevated. My primary care physician then sent me to a surgeon who specializes in prostate surgery. That surgeon ordered an ultrasound test and took a biopsy of my prostate. The ultrasound showed no evidence of cancer, but the biopsy showed that I have a "low-grade" type of cancer. She told me the results of the test and said that surgery would cure me of the cancer. She said that her nurse would call me to discuss scheduling the surgery and the nurse would also go over the "informed consent" form that would tell me about the possible side effects of surgery. The surgeon was nice, gave me her card, and told me to call her anytime if I had questions. She then told me that I could schedule the surgery on my way out of her office, but said there was no need to rush; surgery in the next two weeks would be fine. That comment scared me—get this done in two weeks? I want treatment now.

ME: I understand how hard it is to wait when you have cancer. Many people get frustrated while waiting to decide their best course of action. It does take a significant amount of time to schedule tests and visits with multiple physicians. But, there is absolutely no danger in waiting to make a decision about which treatment you might want until you fully understand the choices you have. There is no need to rush. The optimal way to treat your cancer will not change over the next several months, or perhaps even years. Let's slow down and take the time you need to fully assess your options before deciding.

MR. B.: You mean I have months? Years?

ME: Yes. Prostate cancer, especially the type you have, is slow growing. Some patients with prostate cancer actually choose to forgo treatment and do well for years, even a lifetime, so rushing to a decision would not be good for you. We do not know the optimal timing of any of the treatments for prostate cancer, or any other cancers and chronic conditions. So even though you feel anxious, you are not harming yourself by taking time to learn more about your choices and the consequences of choosing one option over another.

MR. B.: This makes me feel better, a little anyway. It's already been nearly two months since I was first diagnosed, and I was worried that the clock was ticking.

ME: I am glad you are somewhat relieved. Let's move on. What else has happened to you in the last two months?

MR. B.: Well, I called my primary care doctor and told him the surgeon said that the surgery would cure my cancer. I was surprised by my doctor's response; he was not happy. He did not say, "Way to go; now you're on the right path." That was what I wanted and expected to hear after I told him about the surgeon's decision. Instead, my personal physician said that I should not just take one doctor's opinion. He did not suggest a second opinion from a surgeon but instead suggested that I go see an oncologist who specializes in radiation therapy for my type of cancer. I admit I was perplexed by my doctor's suggestion to see another specialist. That recommendation seemed to come out of the blue. I thought I already had gone to the best specialist for my cancer. I thought at the time, "A cancer must be removed, right"? There are no other options, or at least that's what I thought. Now I was being told that other options exist and some other doctor would be weighing in on what treatment might be best. To tell you the truth, this did not make me feel comfortable. Also, this entire time, my primary doctor did not tell me what he thought would be best, at least not until later.

ME: Did you go to the radiation oncologist?

MR. B.: Yes. The radiation oncologist told me that radiation would reduce the chances for some of the side effects of surgery—including pain. What I remember most was that he said that radiation therapy is far less likely to cause impotence, but it may increase the chance of losing my bowel function. He said that he has seen numerous men who opted to not have surgery and instead had radiation therapy. He said that in his experience the men were doing well.

This visit left me more confused. I remember thinking, what does "reduced chance for impotence" and "increased chance of losing bowel function mean"? I asked for more detail and got handed a booklet to read. The booklet was thorough; there were graphs and tables showing the side effects of surgery and radiation. However, the numbers were frightening, and I did not fully understand them, and I have always been good at math.

I called my primary care physician after both of these visits and made an appointment to talk with him about my confusion. He was kind and explained that, unfortunately, there is no best treatment plan. He said he was sorry that I had to go see so many doctors, but he thought I needed to know the options. Then he threw me a curve ball. He said that if he had to decide, he would not do anything but follow along with repeat PSA tests and, perhaps, also have an ultrasound of the prostate repeated on a regular basis.

Now, by my count, I had three options: surgery, radiation, or nothing. I wanted to scream. I wanted to rip my prostate gland from my body with my own hands! I asked my doctor why he ordered the screening test in the first place if he would not have me do anything but follow up without having surgery? Why I am I now the one who must make these choices. I was a healthy man, happy and active, working and playing golf. Why in the world is this happening? These were my thoughts, and my physician noticed my frustration. I could see, also, how upset my doctor was by my reaction. He said that he knew how difficult this was and that I should come to see you. You are the fourth doctor I have seen since finding out that I have cancer. I am not eager for a fourth opinion, but I am totally confused, and the uncertainty and slowness of this process are driving my wife and me crazy. I think I will die of lack of sleep long before this cancer kills me.

ME: I understand your frustration with the many choices. I want you to know that your situation is common. Many patients have seen multiple physicians and have received advice about which treatment to have, but not as much advice about the consequences of the treatment choices.

MR. B.: I did receive a booklet outlining the possible complications with surgery and with radiation. One booklet gave estimates of the likelihoods, but those estimates were described as rare, uncommon, or common. I really don't know what those mean. There are too many options, and I got confused reading the booklet.

ME: Actually, it's good that you have options. The three options offered by the physicians you saw exist because those options, at least some of them, have been tested in groups of patients, and we know something about the good and bad things that may occur with each treatment. Because we can compare, we can tease out the differences in terms of what each treatment offers or takes away for you.

Mr. B., this is important for you to understand, so let me say it again. You have to compare options to know how they are better or worse, so having options is a good thing. Also, without quality studies on outcomes of treatments in groups of patients, treatment choices are just guesses and potentially subject to the whims and biases of individuals or their physicians. A patient making a decision about care should not base that decision on guesses or "my experience tells me" messages. Luckily, for prostate cancer, medical researchers have studied how well patients do if they undergo surgery, or if they chose to just wait and watch the PSA levels over time without undergoing surgery. These two treatments—surgery and no surgery—have been compared head to head; we need now to go over the comparisons. I know you have considered three options: surgery, waiting and watching, or radiation therapy. Since it is difficult to evaluate three options at once, we will start by comparing the only two options ever compared directly.

Unlike the other cases in the chapters that follow, this first case is presented as conversation, because I want you to have the sense of my typical first exchange with a patient. People share similar concerns when they are diagnosed with diseases. Mr. B.'s conversation exposes themes patients face during tough medical decisions. I overemphasize and reiterate these themes in hopes that you will realize the widespread, shared emotions that people have when they are making medical decisions.

12

Beginning to Make a Decision

Mr. B.'s story is not unusual; patients with this cancer have options, and each option carries with it a set of outcomes. Several background medical-care issues need to be understood for this and all decisions. This background information may help you understand why this decision is so difficult and, at the same time, help you understand that there is no best way to treat early stage prostate cancer. The first step to being a better medical decision maker requires knowing about your disease.

Screening for Prostate Cancer

The PSA screening test placed physicians in a quandary between hope and hype. Despite years of use (one estimate suggested that as many as 65 percent of men visiting physicians were screened for prostate cancer in one year), physicians were uncertain if uncovering prostate cancer at an early stage was good for patients. A study from Europe done in the 1960s to 1980s found that the death rate from prostate cancer improved over time despite the fact that treatments for the disease did not change (the most used treatment during the twenty-year period was watchful waiting—only a small number of surgeries were being done during this time period).[1] A study published in *JAMA* found that the reason for this improvement is that the PSA test detected more early-stage prostate cancers than in the past. Because the numbers diagnosed with prostate cancer had gone up, due to earlier detection, but numbers of men dying were the same, the ratio of diagnoses to deaths looked better. Hence, treatment was not advancing care; rather, cancer was being found earlier in the course of disease, so it just looked like things were better.[2]

Chapter 7 discussed study designs and measurement. These two studies, the one study from Europe (reference 1) and the one in *JAMA* (reference 2), were observational studies. Hence, people getting the PSA when it became available may have been different than people getting screened prior to routine use of the PSA test. In other words, the findings of the above studies, as examples, could mean that screening is helpful, or that people getting PSA tests to screen were different people than those who chose other screening procedures. We never know if the cup is half-full or half-empty when we measure outcomes in an observational study. An RCT would be a better study design for measuring the value of a screening test like the PSA. It would be nice to know if people who were, by chance, screened with a PSA test did better in terms of their chance of dying of prostate cancer than those who, by chance, did not get screened. And in fact, at least six RCTs have addressed if screening with a PSA test is useful. For the 387,286 men who consented to be studied in these six RCTs, screening did not improve prostate-cancer-specific mortality.[3] Despite evidence that screening may not reduce the chance of dying of prostate cancer, many men still get a PSA test. Mr. B. said the reason he got the test was that he thought it would prevent any chance of prostate cancer.

The Cancer

Fortunately for some and unfortunately for others, one prostate cancer does not equal another. There are differences in the stage (extent of the disease) at the time of diagnosis, and even how the cells look under the microscope. To make things more complicated, variation in the types of cancer cells between different patients is matched by variation in the different types of cancer cells in the same prostate gland. A mentor of mine once said, "If you have seen one cancer, you have seen one cancer." Some people have prostate cancer and live a full life; some die shortly after diagnosis. Both situations are called "prostate cancer," but they are vastly different. If you become skilled at nothing else from this book, learn that you must fully understand your diagnosis and the percent chances of outcomes, because they foretell your prognosis (not just for cancer but for any disease condition).

Mr. B.'s cancer looked only slightly different than normal under the microscope, and there were two patterns to the abnormal cells. The final report of the microscopic findings classified Mr. B.'s prostate cancer as a "Gleason score of 6." Donald Gleason was a pathologist who in the 1960s devised a scoring system based on the patterns of the cells taken at the time of a prostate gland biopsy. This scoring system has stood the test of time as a prognostic tool. The patterns of the cancer cells from the same prostate gland may vary from well-demarcated, nearly normal-appearing cells, to the wildly bizarre. Gleason's system grades the two most predominant patterns seen on the biopsy specimen. Mr. B.'s score of 6 was a 2-4 pattern (pattern 2 predominates, 4 is less predominate). On the prognosis scale, this is a good pattern to have.

What Options for Prostate Cancer?

For prostate cancer, three main treatment options exist: (1) no treatment other than following with a physician, (2) surgery, or (3) radiation therapy. The treatment that provides the lowest chance of dying of prostate cancer will be preferred—the benefit side. As you now know, the option that may offer the greatest chance of not dying of prostate cancer will also be associated with a greater added chance of harmful outcomes caused by the treatment. Each of these plans is associated with different percent chances of harm, or side effects. Choosing among the three options is a trade-off for a patient.

General Comments about Prostate Cancer (and Cancer in General)

The percent chances of outcomes for prostate cancer are changing so rapidly that it is often difficult to keep up with the changed landscape. A study done ten years ago may provide different estimates for the chances of outcomes than a study done today, even if the treatments, then and now, are the same.

Why aren't prostate cancer outcomes today the same as outcomes in the past? (We are discussing prostate cancer, but this issue about outcomes of care differing over time is true for many, if not all, types of cancer and other chronic diseases, such as heart failure or diabetes.) The reason is that strategies for finding prostate cancer in the first place have advanced— so much so that stage 1 (least extensive) prostate cancer today is different than stage 1 prostate cancer ten to twenty years ago. The advance in detecting cancer earlier means that stage 1 cancer today includes smaller tumors found earlier in their course than those tumors found and classified as stage 1 in the past. If we compare studies about treatments done ten to twenty years ago for stage 1 prostate cancer with studies done today, we are comparing apples and no apples (see chapter 7). The effect of this change in the early detection of cancer is that it makes all treatments look like they are better now than in the past. But this may be a false finding; we are not necessarily getting better at treating cancer; instead, we are treating cancers earlier in their course of disease. In other words, with this earlier detection, we are peering at cancer outcomes from a different point in the course of disease than in the past.

Why are diseases being found earlier in their course? Because we changed how we make the diagnosis. We used to use a "crude" diagnostic tool (a test called the "digital rectal exam"): a physician felt for cancer in the prostate gland. A cancer would have to be quite large before an insensitive tool like a finger could detect it. Now, in contrast, we have a blood test that is more sensitive. "Sensitive" means that smaller cancers, earlier in their course, will be detected: small cancers spill materials into the blood that are found by the precision of the PSA test. This PSA test makes the finger an outdated detection tool.

The reason we are discussing this aspect of screening for cancer is that this advance in earlier detection of cancer may mean we are now finding cancers too early. We may be finding cancer cells so early in their course that they would never disturb our lives. In fact, we may be detecting these cells so early that our body's own defense systems may already have them under control.

Detection of cancer earlier in time and smaller in size may sound good in theory but may not be good in practice. For example, there are two potential implications for an earlier diagnosis by the PSA test. The good implication would be if early diagnosis led to cure. The bad implication would be if early diagnosis led to treatments being proposed too early and before they might help. This is a universal problem with screening for any disease: as we get better at finding diseases earlier in their courses, a greater number of people will be labeled as having the disease. But we may not be helping these labeled persons at all.

You will face this issue all of your life, as tests keep getting more sensitive (genetic tests, for example). The subject of screening for cancer, or other clinical maladies, is so important that a discussion of how to go about making your own choices for screening or preventing illness would fill another book. For now, I am raising your awareness of the potential trade-offs that arise with "testing too early in the course of a disease." A case in chapter 16 touches on the subject of deciding for different types of screening tests.

Treating Prostate Cancer

Mr. B. has stage 1, Gleason's grade 6 prostate cancer. His clinical situation is similar to others: 25 to 45 percent of men who are found to have prostate cancer after a screening test look similar to Mr. B. Fortunately, there is information from randomized controlled trials (RCTs) for Mr. B.'s cancer. In fact, there have been two RCTs that have tested if surgery to remove prostate cancer versus leaving the cancer and the prostate alone would lower the chance of dying of prostate cancer in the future.

In Sweden, Finland, and Iceland, from October 1, 1989, to February 28, 1999, 695 men with prostate cancer localized only in their prostate gland entered into an RCT to test if surgery for prostate cancer reduced the chance of dying of prostate cancer.[4] This study has spawned several follow-up reports, all suggesting an advantage to surgery over doing nothing. In one report, after an eight-year follow-up, 14 percent of men in the do-nothing group died of prostate cancer, and 9 percent died of prostate cancer in the surgery group. Hence, surgery added 5 percent (14 percent – 9 percent) to the chance of not dying of prostate cancer compared with not having surgery. (Note that if surgery was performed and the prostate gland removed entirely, some men still died of prostate cancer.)

Until recently, this study, with its follow-up reports, was the only RCT for early-stage prostate cancer testing surgery versus no surgery, so it is one often used for informed medical decision making, despite some flaws. In this older study, men in the do-nothing group were not offered, for a significant portion of time during the clinical trial, any treatment should they develop local progression (that is, if the cancer spread within the prostate gland). This would not occur today—men who choose to not have surgery would be followed with PSA tests and physician visits, and if the cancer progresses, it would be usual to act on that progression in some way. It would be unusual to do absolutely nothing, even if surgery was not originally done. The difference in how people in the study were treated in the past and how they would be treated now makes it difficult to use that study with patients diagnosed recently. The lack of follow-up treatment for men in this older study who did not have surgical treatment may have made surgery look better than it is; the benefit difference between surgery and no surgery may not be as large as a 5 percent difference.

Newer Information

This criticism of the older study is credible, as shown with the publication of another, more contemporary RCT. This more recent study also enrolled patients who, again, were randomized to surgery or watchful waiting with no surgery. This study was conducted in forty-four Department of Veterans Affairs sites and eight National Cancer Institute sites and enrolled men from 1994 to 2002. The report from this study, published in

2012,[5] described 731 men, one-half getting surgery and one-half getting no surgery, followed for eight to ten years. Unlike the older study, the men in the no-surgery group were offered treatments if the cancer progressed. This recent study, then, had a different study design, and it found different results: instead of 14 percent of men randomized to no surgery dying from prostate cancer in ten years in the older study from Europe, only 8 percent died over a similar time period in the newer study. The difference in the baseline rate of dying, then, without any intervention other than observation, was 6 percent less (14 percent – 8 percent) in the new study. On the surgery side, instead of 9 percent of men dying of prostate cancer in the older study, only 6 percent died—a 3 percent difference. What is the effect of this lower chance of dying for both groups? Since fewer men died of prostate cancer in both groups, the ability of surgery to reduce the percent chance of dying of prostate cancer is less: the difference between the surgery and the no-surgery groups was 8 percent – 6 percent = 2 percent in this recent study, not 5 percent like in the older study.

It is worth repeating why the chance of dying of prostate cancer was lower in both groups in the recent RCT. Remember our discussion above about more sensitive tests: stage 1 cancer in the older study and stage 1 cancer in the newer study were different. In the older study the average PSA score was 13 ng/dl, and in the newer study it was 8 ng/dl (lower is better). Hence, cancers in the more recent study were smaller and detected earlier in the course of the disease (and the PSA test has gotten more sensitive over time). Both treatments, hence, will be associated with better outcomes, and this will lead to smaller chances for finding benefit. This is a common finding in cancer care in general and certainly in prostate cancer. The smaller the percent chance of an outcome occurring in the first place, the less improvement any treatment can offer over another.

Thus, these two important studies show different results. In the more recent study, the 2 percent difference could have occurred by chance alone. In fact, the newer study surmised that radical surgery for localized, low-grade prostate cancer did not statistically significantly lower the chance of dying of prostate cancer and did not extend life expectancy. If surgery is going to benefit a person with prostate cancer, the most it might offer is a 5 percent better chance over eight to ten years of not dying of prostate cancer, based on the older study. This means that, on a *yearly* basis, the best surgery may do is decrease the chance of dying of prostate cancer about 0.5 percent. In the newer study the benefit difference is even smaller—2 percent over ten years, or 0.2 percent per year.

There are also several "subplots" in these studies. First, in men older than sixty-five, there was no difference in the chance of dying of prostate cancer if surgery was assigned versus waiting and watching. Hence, your age at the time of a diagnosis for this clinical problem is an important consideration. Second, the benefit of surgery changed depending on the PSA test result: surgery provided less benefit for men with large PSA elevations. These factors, age and level of the test result, are important facts to individual men. Mr. B.'s PSA level was 5 ng/dl (slightly abnormal), and his age is fifty-five; if surgery is going to provide benefit to someone, Mr. B. is the man.

13

The Flow of Information for
People Making Medical Decisions

The overall process for medical decision making was presented above (see the Decision-Making Checklist at the end of
chapters 2 and 10), but the delivery of the information should
be a carefully constructed conversation. It is best to follow an
unvarying sequence. You might want to ask that information
be presented in uniform steps so you can understand each step
before moving on. Some patients get the concepts of medical
decision making quickly; others do not. One patient, another
engineer, after being told the numbers calculated the trade-off
in his head and told me, "I got this." He then correctly described
the trade-off he faced, left my office in less than thirty minutes,
followed his chosen plan of care, and is doing well years later.
Another patient took hours until he understood his decision.
There is no right or wrong experience. However, I lay out the
information in this specific way to help you think systematically through your decisions:

FLOW OF INFORMATION FOR DECISION MAKING
- You learn information about your disease and the
  options to be discussed.
- You learn about the quality of the clinical information
  for your decision.
- I then show a graph like figure 2 (in chapter 8) for
  a study we will use, but without the numbers filled
  in. After orienting you to the data, I ask you to fill in
  guesses for the percent chances of outcomes. This is
  a crucial part of the process because it tells me your
  level of understanding and sets you up to learn the real
  numbers.

Active participation with the numbers helps you in two ways. First, it allows practice with the format of the presentation. The informing process must be systematic so you can recount accurately and then reflect on the consequences of choosing. The empty table is used to visualize the decision and hold it steady in your mind. The table is a way to show the numbers but also allows you to organize your thinking about what options are available and what outcomes are being compared. Second, I have found that patients are more likely to remember the study numbers if they see them juxtaposed to their own estimates. Patients usually provide incorrect numbers, as the cases below will show. The ultimate test for this process is that patients, by participating, can recount information accurately. With this flow of information, no one has failed, in my experience, to learn his or her numbers.

Mr. B.'s Decision

Let's get back to Mr. B. It took about an hour to talk about the types of studies that would allow him to make meaningful comparisons between surgery and no surgery. After the discussion, I showed him and his wife an empty table of outcomes and treatment options to orient them to the tasks ahead. (Mr. B. and his wife were aware that impotence was a possible harm of surgery, and that was the outcome that concerned him most. I start with just the main benefit and harm outcomes. However, you will see how more outcomes can be addressed.) I then asked him to fill in the table with his best guesses for the percentage of people having the outcomes for both treatment options. His estimates are presented in figure 3.

This is a revealing figure. Mr. B. guessed that 2,000 people had been studied and that surgery reduced the chance of dying of prostate cancer to 0 percent. Also, to him, not doing surgery was a near death sentence (80 percent chance of dying). The trade-off of harm:benefit given his numbers would be a chance of harm (impotence) one-sixteenth the size of the benefit (not dying of prostate cancer) (5 percent : 80 percent = 5/80, or 1:16). If this table was an accurate reflection of Mr. B.'s assumptions, we could understand how Mr. B. might run, not walk, to the operating room. Patients' estimates do reflect their underlying assumptions. In my experience, people overestimate benefit and, conversely, underestimate harm. After Mr. B. filled in his table, I removed his numbers and wrote in the study numbers based on the older RCT discussed above, shown in figure 4. I wrote in one outcome at a time, starting with benefit before harm. You will note in figure 4 that the numbers are not exactly the same

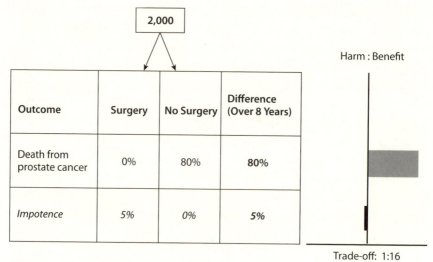

Figure 3. Mr. B.'s Guesses for the Percentage Outcomes for Treatment Options for Prostate Cancer

as those from the reports discussed in chapter 12 (from the European RCT). This is because the numbers in trials are always approximate, and the average numbers are bounded by uncertainty—researchers calculate the average number and then report a 95 percent confidence interval (the range of numbers surrounding the average that reflects a 95 percent chance of what the true number for that study might be). Because there is always uncertainty in the exact numbers for any study, for decision making I recommend using numbers that are easy to remember (such as 10 percent rather than 9 percent)—too much precision is unnecessary.

Although Mr. B. was aware that impotence was a harm of surgery, he was not as aware of the other harmful outcomes. The three harms that have been studied most are impotence, urinary dribbling, and bowel leakage, and all may be experienced for a lifetime. The side effect of surgery that Mr. B. feared was impotence. But the prostate gland is entwined with nerves that serve several important functions nearby: erections, bowel function, and bladder function. The plexus of nerves envelops the prostate gland; removing the gland will affect the nerves. While surgeons are trained to operate in such a way that the nerves are spared, it is impossible to completely assure that the nerves will in fact be spared.

The percent chance of impotence or bladder or bowel leaking varies. In a descriptive study of 5,000 men having surgery, the chance of impotence varied by age, pretreatment sexual function, pretreatment PSA level,

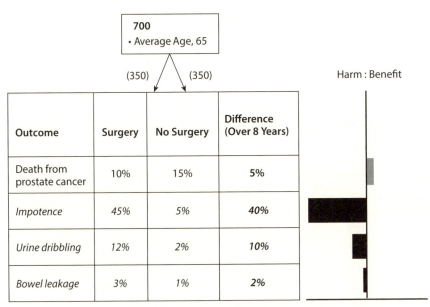

Figure 4. Actual Percentage Outcomes for Treatment Options for Prostate Cancer

and the type of surgery performed.[1] Mr. B.'s percent chance for becoming impotent with surgery, based on this study, was about 45 percent. The chance without surgery is 5 percent (not that doing nothing causes impotence; rather, in time some percentage of men become impotent for reasons other than having surgery).

Figure 4, with actual numbers for the percent chances for the different outcomes with different treatment, shows why this decision is difficult and, again, why only patients should make this choice. It would not be reasonable, or ethical, in my view, to propose surgery, or any other treatment plan, to any patient. Will Mr. B. think that the value to gain from avoiding dying of prostate cancer in eight to ten years is great enough to balance the value to lose from being impotent, dribbling urine, or having bowel leakage, should they occur? In addition, men face harm outcomes sooner after surgery than they would face recurrent cancer if they choose no surgery. There is nothing simple about this sort of decision making, despite a simple process for delineating how the choice may play out in your life.

Let's summarize Mr. B.'s information. (You might want to try this yourself before reading on.) On the benefit side of the decision-making conundrum, the difference in the chance of not dying from prostate cancer between surgery and no surgery for Mr. B. is 5 percent. Remembering our math skills from chapter 8, this means that for an additional single, 100 percent person to not die of prostate cancer eight to ten years from now, twenty men (each getting a 5 percent added chance of not dying) would need to be treated with surgery rather than no surgery (100 percent person ÷ 5 percent chance = 20 people). And this also means that nineteen men would go through surgery without benefit.

There are three outcomes to consider on the harm side of the decision-making conundrum:

- The difference in the chance of being impotent between surgery and no surgery is 40 percent (45 percent – 5 percent). Again, thinking of a single person, for every two to three people who have surgery (100 ÷ 40 percent, with rounding), one person will additionally be impotent. The ratio of harm to benefit for impotence is 40 percent: 5 percent, or 8:1. In other words, about eight men become impotent by the time one additional person does not die of prostate cancer in eight to ten years if surgery is chosen.
- The difference in the chance of having urinary dribbling is 10 percent (12 percent – 2 percent), which means that for every ten people who have surgery, one additional person will have urinary dribbling. The harm:benefit ratio for urinary dribbling is 10 percent : 5 percent, or 2:1. This means that two men will additionally have urinary dribbling by the time one additional person does not die of prostate cancer in eight to ten years.
- The difference in the chance of having bowel leakage is 2 percent (3 percent – 1 percent); for every fifty people who have surgery, one will have bowel leakage. The harm:benefit ratio for bowel leakage is 2 percent to 5 percent, or 1:2.5. This means that, for this one harm, one person will additionally have bowel leakage for every two to three people who do not die of prostate cancer in eight to ten years.

Dealing with the trade-offs for all of these harms can be daunting. I find patients need to mull over the outcomes, the percent differences, and the harm:benefit ratios to fully understand what the numbers mean to them. I also find that patients often make a decision on a single harm-to-benefit outcome balance, but they also do seem to keep in mind the other outcomes. For Mr. B. there are three harm outcomes to balance, and each means something different to his quality of life. You may find that you can only deal with one outcome at a time, and this is perfectly reasonable and, I actually believe, preferable. Some of my patients are on the fence with one trade-off, and then they start to incorporate the other trade-offs. Others seem to intuitively incorporate all balances.

Mr. B.'s Reaction

The numbers surprised Mr. B. He asked me what I would do given those numbers. I replied that I could not make this choice for him—he must come to appreciate whether not dying of prostate cancer in eight to ten years is eight times more value to gain than the value that he would lose should he become impotent, as a first step. Mr. B. said that this was a tough trade-off to understand. And he is correct—it is tough.

To make this trade-off, it is imperative to be fully informed. After the full table is presented and the trade-offs become clear, this is often the moment when patients become aware that they must be their own decision makers. Some patients don't worry about impotence and say benefit, while a smaller added chance, is much greater in terms of the value they will gain than the value they will lose if they become impotent. If this is true, surgery becomes a reasonable personal choice.

Placing personal values on the outcomes of medical treatments is hard work. We don't spend our days thinking, "Is coffee relatively a better drink than water, and if it is better, how much more value does coffee have than water?" But these are just the sorts of trade-offs that the best medical decisions demand. The decision to undergo surgery for prostate cancer is an example of a trade-off common to many medical decisions: we undertake a treatment in hopes of living longer, but in addition, we face an added chance that the treatment may diminish our quality of life. Patients deciding about treatments for cancer face this sort of dilemma every day. For example, deciding for chemotherapy involves balancing the added chance of living longer against the backdrop of toxicity from the chemotherapy agents. If you can learn the process of deciding for this prostate cancer situation, you can apply the process to any of your medical decisions.

Perhaps this example of making a treatment decision for prostate cancer is too dramatic. How about something a bit simpler, like treating high blood pressure? If your blood pressure is elevated, often you are prescribed medications to lower your blood pressure. You may feel well and have no outward or even inward signs that the elevated blood pressure is causing you harm. But if you do not lower your blood pressure to healthy levels, you face an increased chance of having a complication of the elevated blood pressure in the future, such as premature heart disease or kidney failure. The medications you take to lower the chance of adverse outcomes like these may cause side effects. Impotence, for example, is one such harm associated with some of the medicines used to lower blood pressure. Hence, you may have to make balanced judgments about which medication you want to lower your blood pressure. Chapter 15 gives an example of a patient using this process to decide whether to take a second blood-thinning medication when she is already on one. The point is that we can be a part of any decision for our medical care, not just those that entail interventions like surgery with extraordinary lifelong harms like impotence.

Mr. B.'s decision presents an ever-present reminder: there is more to making a decision than just numbers. Deciding how much value there may be to gain versus how much value there may be to lose is *your* work to do. This required balancing is good news, because this is where your life's values intersect with the different percent chances of benefit and harm imposed by different medical tests and treatments. The hard work of balancing the numbers and your values allows you to know the potential consequences of any choice before deciding.

Yet, many patients I have helped with decision making became so overwhelmed by having to make the trade-off between the chance of living longer and the chance of a reduced quality of life that they resorted to wishful thinking as their decision tool. I had a patient who, with his wife, felt that their life was blessed with good fortune and hence that nothing bad could occur from having surgery. This hopeful approach is to be treasured, but it does not stop the biology of chance after a decision is made. That biology of chance supersedes our wishful thinking and even, to be fair, our best-informed decisions. This man and his wife refused to look at numbers. They were respectful but said that I could not help them. They told me "numbers did not matter" because they were individuals and for individuals it was "all or none." They fully expected and trusted that the best would occur. I appreciated their optimism. There was nothing I could do to help them with their choice. True to their values, the man had surgery, and complications followed. He was impotent, had to wear diapers, and needed supplementary surgery to stop his urine from leaking. To some, this would seem a tragic outcome. To his credit, however, when we met later, he was coping. In some sense he made his choice intuitively: for him the surgery was worth the harm that followed. And, if he had chosen surgery after being informed, the same outcomes would have occurred. The difference is in the process or way of going about a decision. The way he went about making his decision made it impossible to realize the potential consequences. When we are facing medical decisions, we must honestly accept that there is biology of chance that pursues us after we have made our choices. Knowing potential consequences before making a choice gives you the best opportunity to align your values for potential gain and loss. Hopefulness and a positive outlook may always be the best when facing a complex medical decision, but hope and a positive outlook are not decision-making tools—they are tools for coping with the consequences of the choices we make.

What Did Mr. B. Decide?

Mr. B. and his wife struggled with Mr. B.'s medical decision. We spent two more sessions together. In those sessions we reviewed the more recent study showing a smaller added chance of benefit and used more optimistic estimates for impotence. Mr. B.'s original plan was surgery, but after our sessions he decided against it. He said that the chance of dying of prostate cancer was small enough that the added chance of not dying in eight to ten years was not worth the chance of being impotent. He said that the benefit was not eight times more valuable than harm. In fact, he said, it was nearly equal in value to him at this point in his life to be able to have sexual relations as it was to not die at some time in the future. Intuitively and relatively, Mr. B. made a choice. So, instead of surgery, he enrolled in a study to test nutritional ways to lower the risk of prostate cancer progressing. He also told me that his wife's view influenced him; this decision, he realized, affected not only his life but also his wife's. He bemoans undergoing the PSA test and says he will never again have an executive physical exam.

Mr. B. is now fifteen years past his screening test and his decision making about prostate cancer treatment. He has stopped getting testing on a yearly basis because, he says, "I hate having to revisit this decision every year." I remind him, however, that not having surgery does not mean doing nothing; he should still follow up with his physician. For Mr. B., to this point, the consequences of his choice have been favorable.

14

Mr. C.

In chapter 10, I introduced two gentlemen. Mr. B. you got to know in the preceding chapters. Mr. C. had nearly identical characteristics of prostate cancer, but he faced different decision-making issues than Mr. B. As far as the cancer's biology is concerned, Mr. C.'s prostate cancer might be confused with Mr. B.'s: the pathology of the tumor was similar and the Gleason score was also 6; Mr. C.'s PSA level was higher, but only by a small amount. A difference was that Mr. C.'s prostate cancer was found in four of the biopsy specimens done by his urologist, as opposed to two for Mr. B. The cancer cells, fortunately, were localized to one side of the gland. Mr. C. was also different than Mr. B. in ways that have nothing to do with having cancer. Mr. C. was older, sixty-five, and had had two heart attacks. These attacks were mild, and he was still active and considered himself to be in good health. Mr. C. was scheduled for surgery despite being advised by his personal physician that radiation may be better. He told a friend about his decision. That friend had seen me in the past and suggested that Mr. C. see me. The friend had faced the same decision and chose radiation therapy, and he told Mr. C. Though Mr. C. was not eager to see me, he relented.

After meeting with Mr. C., I found that he had another situation that differed from Mr. B.'s: Mr. C. was impotent. After his second heart attack, medicines and the stress of recovery left him unable to have sexual relations. Hence, one of the potential harms of surgery was removed. Mr. C. also had different numbers for benefit. As a reminder, Mr. B., at fifty-five years of age, had a 2 to 5 percent added chance of not dying of prostate cancer with surgery. Mr. C. was older, and perhaps surgery would not afford the same potential benefit. Unfortunately, it is unclear whether at his age there is any added chance of not dying of prostate cancer with surgery, because in the randomized controlled trials (RCTs) surgery did not add to the chance of not dying of prostate cancer for older men, and even observational studies do not find benefit in older men. It may be that older men tend to have other maladies besides the prostate cancer that influence their futures more than having the cancer. Scientists call this factor "competing comorbidities." This is a fancy term for a simple idea: no one should undergo a treatment if the benefit of that treatment takes longer to accrue than there is time to accrue it.

This difference in benefit numbers based on a person's age is one of the important reasons that making choices is so personal. Many physicians and patients read a medical paper about a treatment and believe that each person in the study gets the same benefit. This is not true; for patients in a study, some get no benefit, some get some, and some get more. The average number is not the important number—the important number is the one that fits you. Applying the average numeric result to a patient who could never benefit would be reckless patient decision making.

The information for Mr. C. from the RCTs is that patients over the age of sixty-five did not have an added chance of not dying; hence, surgery did not significantly benefit older men. The benefit difference is 0 percent, not 2 percent or 5 percent. One of the critiques of this assertion (that surgery fails to benefit older men) is that the information for this age group is uncertain. The reason for the uncertainty is that not many older men have been studied in clinical trials, so the confidence in the 0 percent estimate of benefit is not strong. In the more recent study described above, for example, of the 731 men in the study, only 242 men who underwent surgery were older than age sixty-five.[1] What can be said to Mr. C. is that, at present, no study provides evidence of benefit for certain. Perhaps future studies will include older men, and our assertion of lack of benefit for older men may be affirmed or refuted. However, presently, we cannot tell men in Mr. C.'s age group that there is a benefit of surgery over doing no surgery.

The reported lack of benefit in older men has led some to suggest that screening may not be helpful in men of Mr. C.'s age.[2] Mr. C. did get screened by his physician during a follow-up exam for his heart disease and now faces the choice for surgery. I talked with Mr. C. after finding out about his impotence and asked him if he feared or worried about any other side effects or harms of surgery. He said he did not know there were

others. I said there were: since the nerves are near the bowel and bladder, some men after surgery will dribble urine and may even have diffi-
culty with controlling bowel functions, necessitating diapers. His face told
me that he was surprised. He and his surgeon had talked only about the
added chance of harm of impotence.

Mr. C.'s decision table was different than Mr. B.'s. For Mr. C.'s guess table,
he thought that the chance of dying of prostate cancer was 10 percent if
surgery was done and 40 percent without surgery (30 percent difference,
or benefit). His estimates for urinary dribbling and bowel dysfunction
were 10 percent and 3 percent, respectively, and for all harms without
surgery, 0 percent. His estimates, like Mr. B.'s, were optimistic for benefit
but closer to being accurate for harms: the actual estimates for his age
group are about 15 percent for urinary problems and 10 percent for bowel
problems. In summary, Mr. C. has no benefit numbers to deal with, only
numbers for harm. On the surface, no decision is needed—surgery can't
help him; it can only hurt him.

When I showed Mr. C. his accurate numbers, he became sullen. I asked
him if he understood, and he remained quiet. When I asked him to repeat
the numbers so I could be sure that he understood what we had been talking about, he refused to repeat the numbers. After what seemed an hour,
but was only a few minutes, I am sure, he told me that he did not believe
that surgery would not benefit him. He did not like the added chance of
dribbling urine, but in this, our first meeting, harm outcomes were not
foremost on his mind—he was upset by the suggestion that there may be
no benefit to surgery. He asked me why anyone would offer surgery if it
did not help and then asked me how, since I was not a surgeon, could I
know surgery does not help.

Mr. C. left our meeting abruptly. I got a call from his urologist, who
was upset with me for showing the data on the benefit of surgery for
men sixty-five or more years of age. He told me I should have used the
average number for benefit rather than the number for older men. The
urologist also said things that I would not repeat in print. I then got a call
from Mr. C.'s friend. The friend was happy, almost giddy, and his mood
contrasted sharply with the urologist's. That friend had advised Mr. C.
to recant his decision for surgery. The friend thought that, after seeing
the real numbers, Mr. C. would alter his decision and not have surgery.
I was not offended that Mr. C. and his surgeon were upset, because often
patients are not told the numbers for consequences, and then can be
unpleasantly surprised when they are.

After a few days, since Mr. C. lived close to me, I decided to go to his home along with the friend. I asked the friend, however, to not advise Mr. C. I reminded the friend that only the patient could make the choice, not a physician or a friend. I know the friend cared, but caring during decision making sometimes means being quiet. Mr. C. invited us into his home, and then the first thing he did was say he was sorry for treating me the way he did. I assured him it was not a problem; I told him that I understood how difficult it would be to make this decision, and that I understood that the urologist had operated many more times than I—he laughed. I told him that all I hoped to do was let him know the best information I could find for him. I brought with me the literature I used to construct his information table so he could see the numbers for himself. He looked at the papers with feigned interest, peering at them like they were foreign objects.

During our visit, Mr. C. said he was scheduled for surgery. He believed in his surgeon and thought that, despite the lack of studies showing certain benefit, studies can be wrong, too. He believed that surgery may make a difference in his life expectancy, and he wanted to avoid any chance of dying of prostate cancer. He also said that he woke up every day thinking of the cancer lurking inside, and he just wanted it out. He thought that removing the prostate gland would ease his mind. Mr. C. believed that removing cancer would be a good outcome regardless of the future. I reminded Mr. C. that the task of choosing options of care during medical decision making is not to count how many people have their prostate glands removed but, instead, to count how many are benefited or harmed by removing it. He said, "I get your point; removing my cancer may not matter to my future at all. I have to think this through a bit more."

Mr. C.'s Decision

Mr. C. went to surgery to remove his prostate gland several weeks after our meeting. I visited him in the hospital, and he did well. I have never seen Mr. C. again.

Mr. C.'s and Mr. B.'s decision-making experiences were different. For Mr. B., benefit was possible from surgery, yet he chose against it. For Mr. C., on the other hand, there was no added chance that he would do better with surgery, and yet he chose surgery. Both men evaluated their own trade-offs—a balance of benefit versus harm, of hope versus knowledge—and made their decision. Both decisions were true for them, were personally correct, because both men knew the consequences of the choices they made and could not deny their hand in making the choice. Both went through an informing process, and, like their results or not, they were responsive to and responsible for learning what may happen to them should they have surgery or other treatments for prostate cancer. The goal of informed decision making is not uniform decisions, but a uniform process of being informed. There is no way to know what individuals will do once they know the consequences of the choices they face, just like there is no way to know what, exactly, will happen as a consequence of that decision. But, once informed, the decision is theirs to make—just as once the decision is made, the consequences are theirs to experience.

Here is a brief, last story of prostate cancer decision making. Mr. and Mrs. Y. went through the process of being informed and made a choice based on their concerns about the quality of the studies done in men with prostate cancer. The studies included no person in their ethnic group. I told them that we had no evidence that ethnicity altered the responses of surgery or any other therapy for the outcomes of early-stage prostate cancer. I could not argue, however, with their assessment; their ethnic group had not been studied. This was enough information for them. They decided to forgo treatments and wait. After an hour of discussion, they chose the path they wanted.

I don't know what to think of this situation. I was not completely comfortable with the encounter. Mr. and Mrs. Y. refused to learn the harm and the benefit numbers because they discounted the value of the information for them in the first place. But Mr. and Mrs. Y. taught me that information in its full extent must be presented to people so they can make choices. By "full extent" I mean that presenting information to patients must include data on the number and types of people included in the study. These pieces of information were important to Mr. and Mrs. Y. As discussed in chapters 5–8 on the science of medical information, measurement errors can occur not only during the conduct of a study but also due to limits imposed by the populations of people being studied. You have the right to a transparent presentation of scientific information, even with and, perhaps more important, because of its possible flaws.

15

Mrs. D.'s Not-So-Dramatic Decision to Make

The choice between surgery and no surgery for prostate cancer is a striking one; balancing the potential to reduce the chance of dying versus the potential added chances of serious complications that last a lifetime with surgery is demanding and taxing. But the process for making a decision for prostate cancer is similar to the process for any medical decision that requires a trade-off, even if the consequence are not so life altering. The crucial concept in medical decision making is the trade-off. The goal of medical decision making is to know if the trade-off is worth it to you.

For some medical decisions, the trade-off balance may be one-sided in terms of the values being traded. Even a vanishingly small chance of benefit for a major valued outcome may overwhelm certain minor inconveniences that are not permanent. An example may be the flu vaccine decision: the benefit side of receiving the vaccine is the small added chance of not getting seriously ill; the harm side is minor in comparison—a sore arm for a day or so, with no long-term harm outcomes. For this type of decision, the value to gain is much greater than the value to loose. Another example is taking an antibiotic for bacterial pneumonia; the benefit outcome for taking antibiotics (saving life) overwhelms the side effects of taking a pill, which are minor in comparison (nausea, for example—I am not saying nausea is minor, just that it is a minor part of the trade-off to something as dramatic as the benefit of treatment if you have pneumonia). Yet, despite the inequality in the values to gain or lose for these sorts of choices, it is still better to follow the process you are learning. This approach applies to making any decision, no matter how uneven the chances of harm and benefit outcomes on each side of the decision equation might be. Let's see how another patient decided about taking or not taking an additional medicine for her clinical malady. The trade-off may be a bit less dramatic than with the prostate cancer decision, but going through our approach helped her make a choice.

Peripheral Arterial Disease

Our arterial system is required to keep us up and running. A perturbation in our arteries may lead to serious consequences. Keeping the arterial road free of bumps, narrows, and holes is a good thing. There are factors that contribute to the arterial system getting clogged. High blood pressure, smoking, aging, and other conditions are associated with narrowing of the arteries. Depending on which part of the arterial system narrows, different clinical conditions occur. For example, heart attacks may occur if the narrowing occurs in the coronary arteries; a person may develop pain in the legs if the narrowing is in arteries there.

Pain in the leg due to narrowed arteries is called "claudication," and a narrowed artery to the leg is called peripheral artery disease (PAD). Besides causing symptoms in the leg, PAD is also associated with other problems with arteries, such as narrowed arteries in the heart or brain. When vessels are narrowed in one part of the body, other clinical conditions related to narrowed vessels tend to happen as well—like birds of a feather. Keeping the arteries open may take a surgical procedure if the narrowing is so severe that blood flow ceases, but most people with PAD do not have this dramatic outcome and so take medicines, such as aspirin, to help them care for their PAD. Aspirin keeps the platelets in our blood less "sticky," and this added fluidity helps keep the blood in a diseased artery flowing. Aspirin is one mainstay for treatment, used to reduce pain and help patients with PAD be less debilitated by the narrowed artery.

But some physicians recommend a second medication be added to aspirin for patients with PAD. The thought may be that, since PAD is a harbinger of other problems, perhaps more medicine may protect not only from PAD but also from strokes or heart attacks. One such medicine is clopidogrel, but there are others that work similarly. Clopidogrel works like aspirin to keep platelets less sticky, which sounds like a good thing. But is adding this second medicine to aspirin worth it? This is an important question for many people. Studies find that as many as 15 percent of people over the age of seventy have PAD. That is a lot of people, so a lot of people may have to decide how many medicines to take for their PAD, just like Mrs. D. had to do.

Mrs. D. and Her Peripheral Artery Disease

Mrs. D. is sixty years old, married, a grandmother, feisty, likes to be in control, and has wonderfully taken care of her diabetes for many years. Her diabetes is "mild," she says, and she never has had problems with maintaining her blood sugar levels. In fact, she tells me, she is not sure she really has diabetes. Nor has she had complications of diabetes. She watches her diet; she takes her medicines regularly and keeps her blood sugar levels in a nearly normal range. She does not take insulin but does take other medicines for her diabetes and tells me that the worst thing about having diabetes is taking the many medicines. Mrs. D. used to smoke and drink alcohol "a bit," but quit both over twenty years ago. She told me she now has no vices other than "high-stakes" (25 cent) bingo.

About two years ago, Mrs. D. noted pain in her legs when she went for vigorous walks. When she would slow down, the pain lessened. But since the pain seemed to come each time she went for a strenuous walk, she decided to see her physician. The physician sent Mrs. D. for tests on her legs that showed that the arteries were narrowed, but not severely enough that surgery would be required. However, afterward Mrs. D. was told to add another medicine to her list: aspirin. She took aspirin as diligently as her other medicines for two years without incident. Now, two years after the diagnosis of PAD, Mrs. D.'s physician sent her to a specialist for another matter and that specialist, in talking with her about her general care, recommended adding clopidogrel to the aspirin. The reason she was given for adding the second medicine was that taking two medicines was "more likely to prevent strokes."

Are Two Medicines Better than One?

Aspirin is commonly used in patients with narrowed vessels, because narrowed vessels are a risk factor for untoward outcomes in the future. In a study of patients with risk factors for stroke due to narrowed arteries, aspirin reduced the chance of a future stroke from 2.5 percent to 2.1 percent compared with not taking aspirin.[1]

Let's review the numbers for this study. The percent chance of having a stroke in the group of patients not taking aspirin is 2.5 percent, and the percent chance in the group of patients taking aspirin is 2.1 percent; 2.5 percent – 2.1 percent equals 0.4 percent, or a 0.4 percent lower chance of having a stoke in the future. How many people would have to be treated with aspirin rather than nothing before a single person benefits? If you divide 100 by 0.4 percent, you get 250; so 250 people would have to take aspirin on a daily basis to have one additional person avoid a stroke. On the flip side, 249 people will take aspirin daily and not benefit from taking the medicine. (I will not talk of the harm side for aspirin because we need to address Mrs. D.'s question first, but certainly there is a greater percent chance of bleeding with aspirin, even if the bleeding might be minor in nature.)

This 0.4 percent chance difference is small, and the confidence in this difference is not strong. One of the reasons for the curtailed confidence, from a scientific point of view, is that the percent chance of a stroke is low even if aspirin is not taken. Hence, a huge number of patients would have to be studied to find, for certain, a lower percent chance of having a stroke at a starting chance for a stroke of 2.5 percent with no treatment at all. This is because the smaller the difference between competing treatments, the more patients we need in the study to be able to find that difference. In other words, a new treatment added to aspirin would have to be remarkably powerful to reduce a small baseline risk for stroke of 2.1 percent already afforded by taking aspirin. It will take tricky scientific work to find if clopidogrel plus aspirin adds to the percent chance of not having a stroke over taking aspirin alone.

The Study Comparing Two Medicines to Just One

In 2006, that tricky scientific work was done: an RCT was conducted to test whether two medicines are better than one for patients with PAD. That study asked whether adding clopidogrel additionally benefited patients already taking aspirin.[2] Like so many other studies, this study was tagged with a catchy name so that it would stand out in memory: the CHARISMA study, for "Clopidogrel for High Atherothrombotic Risk and Ischemic Stabilization, Management, and Avoidance." The potential benefit outcomes measured in the study were lower risk of heart attack, stroke, or dying of any type of cardiovascular cause. In the CHARISMA study, patients were randomized to receive the combination of aspirin plus clopidogrel or just aspirin (and a placebo). The three outcomes were summed to form a single measure, because the researchers knew that each outcome, individually, would occur so infrequently that the study could never recruit enough patients to examine them individually.

This type of outcome measure, combining several outcome events into a single measure, is called a "composite-outcome" measure. Many studies use composite-outcome measures because studies measuring just one outcome might require tens of thousands of patients and dozens of years to complete, making them impractical. The downside, however, and the reason I do not like these studies to help patients decide, is that each of the individual outcomes, now mashed together, may mean something different to quality of life. For example, the value in your life you would lose by suffering a heart attack and the value you would lose by suffering a stroke are likely quite different. Other researchers state that these composite-outcome studies for many of the low-percent-chance outcome events that we face are the best we can do. I don't agree—I think we can do better. But you have to know about this issue for your decision making. The best you can do, at present, is to know when the studies you are using for medical decision making are studies of composite outcomes. For Mrs. D.'s decision, this was the case.

Of the 15,600 patients studied in the CHARISMA trial, those patients taking the combination of aspirin plus clopidogrel had a lower percent chance of having the composite outcome than did patients taking aspirin alone: 6.8 percent versus 7.3 percent; 7.3 percent – 6.8 percent is 0.5 percent added chance of not having one of the three outcome events. So, if this percent difference is correct, 200 people, each getting a 0.5 percent added chance of not having one of the three outcome events, would have to take the combination of aspirin plus clopidogrel to avoid any of these three events from occurring in a single additional person. So, 199 people would take the combination and receive no benefit of adding the second medicine.

Now the harm side: since both medicines affect the platelets, which are responsible, in part, for keeping us from bleeding or stopping bleeding should it occur, taking them both increases the percent chance that a bleeding event will occur. That turned out to be so: the percent chance of a severe bleeding event in patients taking aspirin plus clopidogrel was 1.7 percent, and the percent chance in the aspirin plus placebo group was 1.3 percent; 1.7 percent – 1.3 percent is 0.4 percent added chance of suffering severe bleeding. Hence, for every 250 people who take the combination rather than aspirin alone, one additional person will have severe bleeding. The flip side of the harm discussion is that 249 out of 250 patients will not additionally bleed if they take the second medicine.

Mrs. D. has a trade-off: a 0.5 percent added chance of not having one of three serious outcome events in the future—heart attack, stroke, or dying of cardiovascular disease—and a 0.4 percent added chance of severe bleeding. These numbers are pretty close to being the same, and to make it easier on Mrs. D., I used 0.5 percent for both the benefit and harm outcome events. Again, we do not need undue precision in the clinical decision-making process.

Mrs. D.'s Decision Making

Mrs. D. and I talked about her options, and I asked her level of understanding. She knew of the potential added risk of severe bleeding, and she was also concerned about the added cost of the second medicine. Mrs. D. did not know her chances of having one of the three outcomes. Again, we started with an empty table, and she added her best guesses: a 5 percent chance of one of the three outcomes on two medicines, and 20 percent with just aspirin. The difference for her estimate was 15 percent (20 percent – 5 percent) benefit for taking two medicines. For severe bleeding, Mrs. D. thought the two would increase her chances from 10 percent on aspirin to 12 percent on both, or 2 percent harm (12 percent – 10 percent). She was astutely aware of the trade-off and correctly gave me the harm:benefit ratio for her guesses; benefit was over seven times that of harm (2 percent : 15 percent, or about 1:7). She told me, then, that the value to gain from avoiding a heart attack, stroke, or dying is much greater than the value to lose with bleeding because the bleeding did not necessarily lead to serious clinical outcomes like dying; most are bleeding episodes requiring transfusion support. At this point, she planned to take the second medicine. Given her estimates of benefit and harm, and hence the trade-off, this makes sense.

I then showed Mrs. D. the study numbers (figure 5). Note that the difference in the bottom row is 0.4 percent for harm, but since the numbers are small and similar in amount, I presented Mrs. D. 0.5 percent for both. I violate my own rules in this figure: in most cases I do not use decimal points but instead round up or down to whole numbers that are easier to use and remember. However, in this case, if I rounded up and down, there would be no difference for benefit. Hence, this presentation is a "best-case" situation for two medicines. If Mrs. D. would not chose two medicines with this small difference, then presenting the rounded, 0 percent number would not be needed. Mrs. D. was surprised, and elated, by the numbers. She was able to recount the numbers clearly and was able to calculate the added chances of benefit and harm. She noted immediately that her percent chance of having serious outcomes was less than she thought. She thought there was a 20 percent chance, and when she saw her real chances, she started to change her mind about taking the second medicine. She walked to the information table on a flip-board easel in my

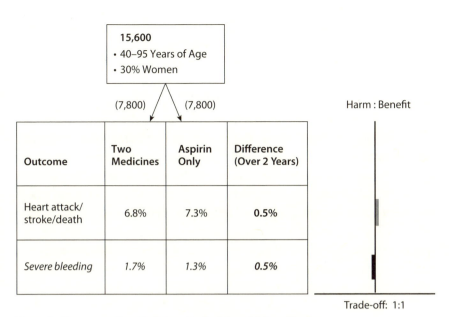

Figure 5. One versus Two Medicines for Peripheral Artery Disease

office and stared for a moment. I then asked her what this meant to her. She told me that a heart attack, a stroke, and dying of a cardiovascular event were scary events. Bleeding to her seemed more a nuisance because bleeding would not affect her life like the other events, given most severe bleeding events were not life threatening. She also noted that the differences were small. She said, almost off-handedly, that she thought these powerful medicines would do more good than they do. I told her that the main problem from the standpoint of the science is that most people do well anyway, so it is hard to determine if any added medicine is truly better. I then reminded her of the other way of looking at the information: "It would take about 200 people taking the combination treatment before an additional person would not have one of the three events. That means that 199 of 200 will get no benefit." And I pointed out that a similar thing could be said about the added chance of severe bleeding complications: about 200 people would have to take the combination before one more patient would have a severe, potentially life-threatening bleeding episode. Hence, 199 of 200 people would not additionally face a severe bleeding complication from the combination. This is a nearly equal-percent-chance trade-off of benefit and harm, and all she had to do was figure out if she would gain more in her life's quality for avoiding any of the three outcomes than she would lose having an episode of severe bleeding. If she would gain more, it would be reasonable to take the combination. If she would not, or could not tell, it would be reasonable to stay with aspirin alone. Then she asked me a great question: "Am I in a lower chance group or a higher chance group for having one of the three outcomes?"

This is an important question. In the CHARISMA study, some clinical factors changed the harm:benefit trade-off. For patients with multiple risk factors, adding the second medicine made things worse: 6.6 percent taking the combination had serious outcomes versus 5.5 percent not taking it, a 1 percent added chance of one of the three outcomes. Each person's decision-making experience will involve nuances in harm and benefit numbers based on variable, personal characteristics—that's the reason that you must go over information with your physician: you must be sure the data fits you. Mrs. D. did not have the factors that would make adding the second treatment more harmful, so we could be somewhat confident that there may be some benefit. In fact, I said that for those patients with clinical symptoms such as pain when walking, like her, the added chance of benefit might be 1 percent, not 0.5 percent. I showed her the study, gave her a copy, and made sure she understood the time frame for the study (about twenty-eight months). So, to potentially have the added chance of benefit, she would have to take the combination for at least two and a half years.

Mrs. D.'s Decision

When Mrs. D. was leaving, she asked for her information, so I gave her the figure from the easel. Despite Mrs. D.'s desires for control of her medical care, she asked me, like many do, "What would you do?" I told her that it would not be fair for me to influence her decision—only she should choose. She politely grumbled at me, called me a coward, and said she would let me know what she decided.

She took her information to her primary physician's office. Her physician is a friend of mine and had referred Mrs. D. to me, because he knows that she is a stickler for her care and can even be bossy if she wants something. Her primary care physician looked at the tables and later told me that he was also surprised by the small difference in the percent chance of added benefit for adding a second medication. I am not sure what conversation then took place between Mrs. D. and her physician, but later she told me that their attitudes changed based on the information.

Mrs. D. decided not to take the second blood-thinning medication despite the greater value to gain from avoiding a heart attack, stroke, or dying. She announced, "The numbers are small; it does not seem to matter that much what I do, and if it doesn't matter that much, I rather not take any more medicines." I saw Mrs. D. three more times to review other medicines. She said that if all of her medicines were doing so little for her, then perhaps she should stop others, too. By the end of our last visit, Mrs. D. had stopped other medicines she had been taking and told me that she is contemplating even stopping aspirin, as she is uneasy about the size of the benefit for taking aspirin daily. She reiterated that the small differences in the number of people having the outcome events between taking the combination versus taking only aspirin was the main factor in her decision making. She had had the internal belief that most of her medicines would have large and positive effects on her life history. When she saw how small some of the differences were, she did not think the medicines were worth the effort to take them. But other patients I have consulted with on this issue have chosen otherwise.

So, the approach of balancing the added chance of benefit and the added chance of harm from your personal perspective will help you be informed, even about your medicines. Perhaps the outcomes of decisions for or against taking medicines may not be as dramatic as those for surgery for prostate cancer, for example, but following the same approach to making choices will allow you to slow down and contemplate the potential effects of your choice. For Mrs. D., the numbers mattered. She is now more informed, but this has led to one, unanticipated, adverse side effect: she is now even bossier about her medical care.

16

Using the Informed Medical-Decision-Making Process for Tests

When I began writing this book, my goal was to help you learn to participate in your decisions about treatments, or at least make you aware of how you can become an active participant in your care. Patients I had consulted with in the past (before the last two to three years) came to decide about a treatment. This was because their diagnosis had already been made and their malady uncovered. I examine test results for patients I see, but I have had no hand in the decisions for which tests were used to make a diagnosis.

But ignoring informed decision making for making a diagnosis was shortsighted on my part. As I have been writing this book, the types of questions I am asked have changed. I am not sure why—perhaps it is serendipity, but I don't think so. Patients have started coming for help with questions about tests rather than treatments; for example, one came to discuss if he should undergo screening for prostate cancer with the PSA test, one came to discuss screening for lung cancer with the CAT scan (see discussion in chapter 8), and one came to decide if she should have a magnetic resonance imaging (MRI) scan rather than a mammogram to screen for breast cancer. (Screening means that you have no inkling that something is amiss, so the test is done to find a disease when it is clinically unapparent.)

I love the challenge of making a diagnosis. I prefer making diagnoses with only clinical information and a few necessary tests, and eschew the trend in performing an excessive number of costly diagnostic tests. My love of diagnosis is likely one reason I studied the disciplines of internal medicine and oncology: they involve making diagnoses as much as treating people once a diagnosis is made. If I wanted to be an excellent diagnostician, I knew I would have to study how to best manage diagnostic tests. For example, a diagnosis may be so evident in a patient that getting an imperfect test for that already likely diagnosis may lead one astray rather than toward the right choice of action. That's because tests are not perfect—they can give false positive and false negative results.

Given my love of diagnostic thinking, I was fortunate to be involved in a study from the National Institutes of Health on how to improve diagnosis decision making. Our research team was charged with defining "diagnosis mistakes" and then finding ways to reduce those mistakes. Our study was an exploration of the imperfections of diagnostic tests and human judgment.

Tests fail in two major ways:

1. The test result says you may have a disease when you do not.
2. The test result says you do not have a disease when you do.

In the first situation, the test result is called a false positive. Test results are either normal or abnormal, whether they are clinical, laboratory, or radiologic tests. But an abnormality on a test does not mean that a specific condition is present. An abnormal test result implies you may have a disease; if in truth the disease is not there, the test's result is a false positive. You saw an example of this in chapter 8 with the study of a CAT scan looking for cancer in people who smoke or have smoked. A CAT scan result can be abnormal if cancer is present, or it can be abnormal for other reasons. The problem for decision makers is that finding out if the abnormal test result is true or not may require dangerous or costly procedures.

If, on the other hand, the test result says you do not have a disease when you do (the second of the two situations above), the result is called a false negative. This means the test result says you are fine but in truth the disease is present. The false positive and false negative results of imperfect tests plague all clinicians and patients, but the reality is that no test is as good as we think it is. Most people, including physicians, put too much faith in tests. Most tests used in diagnosis are not "gold standard" tests; whose results define the diseases. But gold-standard tests may be unavailable, dangerous, or costly, so "screening" or preliminary tests are used. The patients I mentioned at the beginning of this chapter were seeking help for decisions regarding screening tests, which are not perfect tests. For example, the PSA test used for screening for prostate cancer may be elevated in conditions other than cancer; the CAT scan for lung cancer may find an abnormality that is not cancer; both the MRI and the mammogram may show that cancer might be there when it is not; and any of these might miss cancer altogether.

I am delighted that patients are coming more often to discuss diagnostic test decisions; they have alerted me to acknowledge that the process for deciding about diagnostic tests is actually the same as the process for deciding about treatments.

How Are Test and Treatment Decisions Similar?

There are far more similarities between test and treatment decisions than might seem evident at first blush. First, for both diagnostic testing and treatment decisions, options exist. Since the option that is better for one aspect of your health is also more harmful to other aspects, you will have to make trade-offs: a test that is better at finding a specific disease is also worse at falsely identifying people as having that specific disease when it is not there. In other words, as a test dials up the chance of finding a disease (gets more "sensitive"), the false-positive percentage goes up at the same time. Hence, the added percent chance that a correct diagnosis will be made by one test versus another (benefit) must be balanced against the added percent chance that the test will say the disease is present when it is not (harm). Sounds like treatment decision making, doesn't it?

Decisions for tests, then, like decisions for treatments, require you to make a judgment about how much value you may gain for an added chance of a correct diagnosis versus how much value you may lose for the added chance that you will experience the harm of a false positive.

How Do Treatment and Diagnosis Decisions Differ?

Conceptually and practically, diagnosis and treatment decisions require trade-offs. However, the outcomes being measured and compared are different. For treatment decision making, the disease is known and the outcomes are the consequences of the disease condition. In diagnostic testing decisions, alternatively, the outcome is a diagnosis of the disease itself. The benefit of one test versus another is in more likely making a correct diagnosis of a specific disease. The harm of one test versus another is more misdiagnosis of normal people. Like treatment decision making, test decision making is a comparison, but the outcomes being compared differ.

The best way to illustrate decision making for diagnostic tests is to show how one of my patients decided which test to use to screen for breast cancer. She came to see me to discuss if she should undergo another MRI after a first found areas in her breast that looked like they might be cancer. She was accustomed to having a mammogram, but as the story unfolds below, an MRI was ordered instead. The MRI test found "calcified" areas, not seen on previous mammograms, which required biopsies to see if cancer was present; she had had two biopsy procedures, because there were multiple suspicious areas. The biopsies revealed normal tissue. Now, her physician was asking for a second MRI, and she wondered if she should instead just have a mammogram. She did not want to miss cancer, but the worry and costs of the biopsies and MRI tests were wearing on her. She was asking an interesting question: is the MRI better at finding cancer than the mammogram for Mrs. E?

Breast Cancer Screening

Screening for breast cancer is a complex, controversial, and emotional clinical situation. A 2009 guideline produced by the U.S. Preventive Services Task Force, a group that examines evidence for and against medical tests and treatments, recommended that "routine" mammograms for women over forty but less than fifty years of age should not be encouraged; instead, mammography should be chosen by a woman based on her personal preferences for screening outcomes.[1] This guideline says what should be said in every guideline: the decision for or against screening, or any test or treatment, should be a patient's choice. Knowing the numbers for harm and benefit helps us make better choices. Many feel the added chance of benefit of early detection of breast cancer is worth the added chance that biopsies and other tests may have to be done just to find out that cancer was not there in the first place. Since a trade-off exists, individuals should decide.

However, this guideline caused an outcry among both the public and medical care providers, in my view by those who believe mammograms should be done in all women (again, population decision making rather than individuals making their choices). Putting this controversy aside for a moment, it is my experience that women are used to routine mammograms and have continued to have them despite changes in recommendations. Women are acting as if the recommendations didn't change: screen routinely. In fact, women with decisions about breast cancer screening that come to see me do not ask if screening should be done. Instead, they ask *which* screening test they should choose. The newer screening modalities include computer-aided diagnosis, better mammography films or digital exams, ultrasound, and MRI. The question about which one to use is the question posed by Mrs. E.

Mrs. E. and Her MRI

Mrs. E. is forty-five years old and self-identifies as a health "nut." I asked her what that meant, and she stated that she constantly reads the medical news to keep up on the latest items in medicine, runs every day, eats only organic foods, drinks wine in moderation, makes sure she does not gain an ounce of fat, has never smoked (anything, she winked), and never missed a yearly checkup visit with her physician. She says that she watches the medical shows on television to make sure those physicians get things right. As part of her yearly visits, she has a mammogram—four to date and all normal. After our discussion, I gently agreed that she was a health nut.

Her physician of many years retired. On the first visit to her new physician, Mrs. E. mentioned that it was time for her yearly mammogram. The new physician, however, had just examined Mrs. E.'s breasts and noted thickened breast tissue on both sides. The physician told Mrs. E. that some women have "dense" breast tissue, and because of the density, in her case an MRI of the breast is better for screening for cancer than a mammogram. Mrs. E. had just read about the MRI of the breast and appreciated that her new physician was up on the latest developments. Mrs. E. agreed to the MRI rather than undergo her routine mammogram.

The MRI

The MRI is one of those tests that may find cancer more often than a mammogram when cancer is present. However, the MRI, like all more sensitive tests, also falsely identifies more normal people as potentially having cancer. ("Sensitive" in this context means the proportion of patients with the disease picked up by the test. For example, a test that is 100 percent sensitive finds all disease; a test that is 50 percent sensitive misses the disease half the time.) The decision to screen with an MRI rather than a mammogram is an example of how a test that is better at detecting disease also carries the added harm of being worse at telling normal people they may have the disease—more false positives. Because of the higher percent chance of falsely worrying women without cancer, the MRI has been reserved for situations in which the chance of having cancer of the breast in the first place is higher than usual.

There are several situations that increase the lifetime risk of breast cancer. For example, some gene mutations increase the likelihood of future cancers; when these mutations are present, the lifetime chance of developing breast cancer may be as high as 60 percent, or even higher if other mutations are also present. Clinical factors can also alter the lifetime risk of having breast cancer, such as a family history of breast cancer, or age. For women with these genes and adverse clinical factors, a more "sensitive" way to find cancer at screening may be needed.

In 2004, nearly 2,000 women with a higher lifetime risk of getting breast cancer, based on genetic testing and family history, entered a study in which they underwent both a mammogram and an MRI.[2] It was imperative that each woman have both tests, because the tests can then be directly compared for each woman in the study. Fifty of the nearly 2,000 women in this study, about 2 percent, were ultimately found to have breast cancer during the two years of the study. This is a high percentage for a screening study, you will see, and reflects the higher risk of the population being studied. The study followed a strict protocol so that the two tests could be accurately compared for the difference in the number of cancers detected. The researchers were successful in making sure that the radiologists reading the mammogram and the MRI had no knowledge of the other test's findings. This removed some bias from interpreting the test results.

Of the fifty women with breast cancer, mammography detected about 40 percent (sensitivity of the test is 40 percent, meaning the test found 20 of the 50 cancers but missed 60 percent, or 30 out of 50), and the MRI picked up about 70 percent (a sensitivity of 70 percent—the test found 35 of the cancers but missed 30 percent, or 15 out of 50). Neither test was perfect, but the MRI found more of the existing cancers. The MRI, however, falsely said that cancer might be there when it wasn't at a higher percent chance than the mammogram: it falsely identified about 200 of the nearly 2,000 (10 percent) women: the mammogram, about 100 women (5 percent).

Another difference between treatment and diagnosis decision making is that, in treatment decision making, you compare the percentages of outcomes caused by disease for all options. This is because the proportion of the population with the disease is 100 percent for all treatment options. In contrast, in diagnosis decision making not everyone has the disease at the time of the test, or, most important, the same chance of having the disease in the first place. So, the chances of true and false test results are explainable only in the context of the chance of having the disease in the first place. If the chance of having the disease in the first place is 0 percent, then comparing a test that is 100 percent sensitive to a test that is 50 percent sensitive for finding a disease is meaningless.

Table 2. Mammogram versus MRI for Women of Higher Risk of Having Breast Cancer *(Italics Indicate Harm)*

	MAMMOGRAM	MRI	DIFFERENCE
	• Finds 40 percent of cancers.	• Finds 70 percent of cancers.	• Additional number with cancer found (benefit).
	• Falsely says 5 percent have cancer when they do not.	*• Falsely says 10 percent have cancer when they do not.*	*• Added number without cancer told they might have cancer (harm).*
50 women with cancer	20 found	35 found	Additional 15 women found by MRI
About 2,000 women with no cancer	*100 falsely suspected to have cancer*	*200 falsely suspected to have cancer*	*Additional 100 false positives from MRI*

A test that finds 50 percent of diseased people will find 10 if 20 are diseased and 100 if 200 are diseased. For that reason, with diagnosis decision making, the outcome measure is not a percentage but the number of people with the disease and the number without. The compared differences, then, are not the percentages of outcomes caused by disease or treatments. Rather, we compare the number of people correctly identified (benefit: true positives, true negatives) versus falsely identified (harm: false positives, false negatives) out of those with and without the disease in the first place. You will soon see this idea play out for Mrs. E.

Table 2 summarizes the numbers for the study between mammogram and MRI for higher risk women. (I simplified the numbers so you can focus on the process of decision making.) As in treatment decision making, a trade-off is required. Of the 50 women with cancer, the MRI detects 15 more women with the disease than the mammogram, but it falsely identifies approximately 100 more women of the nearly 2,000 without cancer. The harm:benefit trade-off for women at higher than normal risk of having breast cancer is 100:15, or 7:1. This means that harm is seven times more likely than benefit; seven normal women will be falsely identified for every one additional person correctly diagnosed if the MRI is used rather than the mammogram. Another way to look at test trade-offs is to note that, for every eight women with test results that are abnormal, seven of those test results are wrong. The value to gain from finding an additional cancer with the MRI rather than the mammogram in this population of women must be at least seven times greater than the value to lose while waiting to find out if the cancer is there when it is not.

Some women tell me that this worry while waiting is so taxing that they consider forgoing all screening tests. Others say that finding cancer is far more important than the worry or effort required to find out cancer is not there. This example, then, shows how diagnosis decision making and treatment decision making are similar. Since a trade-off of harm:benefit exists, your values must play a part in your choice. Your evaluation of this issue will, of course, depend on the benefit of early detection in terms of reducing your chance of dying of breast cancer in the future. It is not enough to just think about making a diagnosis; you must also think about what making the diagnosis means for your future life.

Unfortunately, this is still a difficult and unresolved issue for many types of cancers found at screening. For some of the types of cancer detected at screening, there is a benefit for early diagnosis, but for others finding the cancer early may not affect your life. This is called "overdiagnosis", and it occurs commonly when screening tests become better able to detect disease at the expense of false detection in normal people. Such may be the case for breast cancer. An RCT with women screened for breast cancer with twenty-five years of follow-up was published in 2014 in the *British Medical Journal*.[3] This study documents how difficult it is to determine if screening for early breast cancer is worthwhile from a benefit standpoint. Nearly 90,000 women were randomized to screening or not. The screening was conducted during a five-year period at the beginning of the study. More women in the screening part of the study were found to have breast cancer (666 with more-routine screening; 524 with less-routine screening). Over the five years, then, only about 1 percent had cancer (much lower than the 2 percent over two years in the high-risk group described above). Regarding death from breast cancer by the end of the study, 500 women randomized to the screening arm died, and 505 randomized to the no-screening arm died. Thus, the mortality from breast cancer was essentially the same for the two screening strategies. The choice to be screened for breast cancer is complex due to the uncertainty of benefit—some studies show a small benefit, and others don't. This is why you are the one most equipped to deal with this uncertainty from your personal perspective. Patients should make decisions about how they would like to be screened for diseases.

But What about Mrs. E.'s Risk?

Mrs. E. is not at higher than usual risk of having breast cancer. She has no family history of breast cancer and does not have genes that would lead to a higher risk. The only concern, on the part of her physician, was that Mrs. E.'s breasts were "dense." I am not sure what this meant to her physician, but it likely meant that the physician noticed thickened and irregular breast tissue. This is a reasonable assumption because Mrs. E. is a thin woman with little body fat. Noting thickened tissue on a physical exam, however, does not mean that Mrs. E.'s risk is higher due to dense breast tissue. In fact, studies suggest that breast exams by palpation have a low chance of finding cancer and a high chance of finding something that is not cancer. A "dense" breast, then, is difficult to define and therefore difficult to reliably measure.

So, why is the "density" of the breast an issue in the first place? Well, as the breast tissue becomes denser, the mammogram becomes less able to find cancer. Hence, some physicians recommend MRI exams for women with dense breasts, like in Mrs. E.'s presumed situation. But density is not really defined by the physician's hands—radiologists grade the density of breast tissue *after* a mammogram; Mrs. B.'s mammograms returned a density rating of normal. The density grading system goes from low to high, and some physicians and researchers have suggested that an MRI may be better than a mammogram for screening in women with denser breasts. This is an unresolved research issue, however, so there is no certainty. In denser breasts, all screening tests may be less able to discern superfluous from suspicious abnormalities.

However, a study published in 2012 will help us estimate the trade-off for Mrs. E.: over 2,800 women deemed to have a higher than usual risk of having breast cancer in their lifetime were given three rounds of screening for breast cancer, and each round included a mammogram and an ultrasound examination.[4] After the third round of dual screening, some women underwent an MRI. Thus, this study was looking for the incremental increase in finding breast cancer over three full years of screening under three conditions of screening tests: mammogram, ultrasound, and MRI.

The way the researchers defined higher risk for this study was different than how the risk was defined in a study from the Netherlands of high-risk women (presented above). In this study, women were considered to have higher risk if they had dense breasts graded on a mammogram by a radiologist and, in addition, had at least one other risk factor, like a history of breast cancer in the family. After the three rounds of screening, some women agreed to have an MRI. Unfortunately, in this study not all the women had all tests. In fact, of the nearly 1,700 women who could have had the MRI at the end of the third screening cycle of mammogram and ultrasound, only 612 women chose to have one. When the entire eligible population is not included when measuring the outcome of a study, the best we can do is make a best-guess estimate—some uncertainty will remain. Remember the poll about presidential hopefuls from a previous chapter? The same situation exists with this study; not all women were included in measurement.

And to make matters more complex for Mrs. E., her personal history does not match the personal histories of the women in this latter study. Her breasts were not the density required to be included in the study (her mammograms were graded as low density, in contrast to her physician's examination), and she has no personal or family history of breast cancer. Her lifetime risk of breast cancer will be lower than for the women in the study. Mrs. E.'s evidence table will also be different than table 2 presented above for women at high risk (in which 2 percent of women were found to have breast cancer): Mrs. E.'s risk will be closer to the risk found in the second study of three cycles of screening with mammogram and ultrasound, followed by MRI. After the MRI, breast cancer was found in about 4 of 1,000 women. This 4 in 1,000 estimate of prevalence would likely be higher than the estimate for the prevalence of cancer for Mrs. E, because her previous mammograms were normal and not graded as dense. However, 4 in 1,000 is a reasonable place to start her decision-making process, because if she would choose to forgo an MRI based on this higher risk estimate, she certainly would not want the MRI at a lower risk.

This last comment requires a bit more discussion. In informed decision making, it is sometimes necessary to vary between high-risk and low-risk numbers when a single best number is uncertain for an individual patient. When you have to choose among estimates for the baseline percent chances of disease, or benefits and harms of testing or treating, it may help to set up a best-case/worst-case scenario. This is possible, and even ideal, because often estimates for outcomes of your care differ based on your personal characteristics, clinical conditions, or differences in study findings. If you feel strongly about your decision with worst-case estimates, you may be more comfortable with your choice. For Mrs. E., her decision for choosing either a mammogram or an MRI would be biased toward the MRI with estimates for disease prevalence that are higher in the

Table 3. Mammogram versus MRI for Women of Lower Risk of Having Breast Cancer
(Italics Indicate Harm)

	MAMMOGRAM	MRI	DIFFERENCE
	• Finds 40 percent of cancers.	• Finds 70 percent of cancers.	• Additional number with cancer found (benefit).
	• *Falsely says 5 percent have cancer when they do not.*	• *Falsely says 10 percent have cancer when they do not.*	• *Additional number without cancer told they might have cancer (harm).*
4 women with cancer	*2 found*	*4 found*	*Additional 2 found by MRI*
1,000 women with no cancer	*50 falsely suspected to have cancer*	*100 falsely suspected to have cancer*	*Additional 50 false positives from MRI*

first place. (This makes some sense because the more likely the disease, the more we want to make sure we find that disease.) If Mrs. E. chooses to have the mammogram test when the "deck is stacked" for MRI due to higher risk, she can be more sure that her decision is the best one for her.

Mrs. E.'s Decision Making

I told Mrs. E. of the studies discussed above and explained potential problems with knowing her exact estimates for having cancer. We then went through the numbers for the added diagnostic yield of the MRI for women at low risk for breast cancer, which was her situation. Table 3 shows the evidence.

For the study of higher-risk women (50 in about 2,000, in table 2), the ratio of false identification to true detection was 7:1. For the study of women more like Mrs. E., however, the numbers change in table 3. Since fewer cancers are likely in the first place, the difference in the number of cancers detected between the two compared tests will be smaller. In Mrs. E.'s situation, 50 additional women will be told they might have cancer when they do not, and 2 additional women with cancer will be additionally detected with an MRI, so the harm:benefit ratio is 50:2, or 25:1. In other words, for every 1 additional person who is accurately identified as having cancer, 25 will experience a false alarm (or, if preferred, for every 26 positive tests, 1 will be a true positive and 25 will be false positives).

Mrs. E. asked me if her risk was really 4 in 1,000. (In her best-guess table, she had estimated her risk as 1 in 100, or 1 percent). She was relieved to see that her risk might be that low, and I reminded her that perhaps her risk was even lower, but if that were true, there would be an even greater number of extra women who will have a false alarm for every woman who has cancer found by having an MRI rather than a mammogram. I asked her if she understood what I meant, and she said, "I got it." I then told her that we could go through the table again with a risk of 4 in 10,000 instead of 4 in 1,000, or even with a higher chance, like patients with risk factors. I then showed her the table for the high-risk women (table 2). I said this study would not fit her, but it would be the worst case I could think of for her. She said we did not need to go over the information. In fact, she even noted that if her risk were 4 in 10,000 instead of 4 in 1,000, 250 women would have a false alarm for every one cancer additionally found—that since 10,000 is ten times as much as 1,000, the number of false alarms would have to go up by the same ratio of 10.

I was pleased she could understand her trade-off and the uncertainty of the numbers. As you can see from Mrs. E.'s example, the trade-off of an additional person detected versus the additional people falsely identified depends on the underlying risk for the person being tested. This is why there is no best test under all conditions for all diseases. Patients will vary in their percent chances of having a disease. Hence, the values to gain or lose for finding any disease in question versus being falsely alarmed about that disease when it is not present would vary. This means that you can and must participate in medical decision making about the tests recommended for you. Your personal preferences will influence the choice of what test is best for you.

Mrs. E.'s Decision

Mrs. E. canceled the MRI and went back to a yearly mammogram for screening. Her subsequent mammograms have been normal. Using the MRI without full consideration of the possible harms of false detection caught Mrs. E. in a trap: the balance between better detection and the added chance of false findings on the MRI was not twenty-five, or even seven times more valuable to her. You may feel differently.

Mrs. E. had other insights. The MRI was costly: she said she paid over $1,000 out of pocket (above the costs paid by insurance), and biopsies added more personal expense. The amount she had spent exceeded the usual costs of screening (she told me it was nearly the amount she paid for a year of her son's college's tuition). Mrs. E. subsequently fully learned the process of medical decision making and became a teacher in a class of mine about patients' choices. She especially helped teach about making decisions for diagnostic tests. She did not like that she started down this costly and, for her, worrisome path with the MRI and wanted others to know of her experience.

17

What If There Is No Reliable Information?

Three stories follow that demonstrate that decisions do occur despite lack of information from sound science. These stories do *not*, however, in my view, show how decisions should be made when information is lacking, but I will leave that judgment to you after I have made my argument.

Story 1

In the last year, three women have asked for help to decide if they should have bilateral mastectomies (both breasts removed) after finding they had ductal carcinoma in situ (DCIS) in one breast. These women were educated professionals; physicians for two of the women broached the subject, but the third woman asked her physician to schedule the mastectomies. All women felt they wanted both breasts removed in order to remove, in concert, worry brought about by more follow-up testing in their futures. All felt they were sitting on a ticking time bomb, and they wanted any future chance of cancer gone.

DCIS is a specific type of breast cancer diagnosis, one of many. It used to be uncommon, but since the introduction of screening mammography, nearly one in five women with breast cancer is diagnosed with this type. DCIS is not an aggressive type, and a woman diagnosed with DCIS will have a low chance of the cancer coming back or causing death (only 1–2 percent in a lifetime). Hence, life expectancy with DCIS is nearly normal.

Two main surgical options for treating DCIS have been proposed. Unilateral (one breast only) mastectomy, the most studied option, involves removing the entire breast. A lumpectomy, which involves removing only the site of cancer within the breast, not the entire breast, and is followed by radiation therapy, is a more conservative alternative that has not been studied head to head with mastectomy for DCIS. And bilateral mastectomy for DCIS has never been studied—in fact, it has been limited to women with high-risk cancers, such as those with specific genetic abnormalities. Even in those situations RCTs are lacking, and most certainly so for DCIS. So, the potential for benefit for bilateral mastectomy versus unilateral mastectomy is unknown, or 0 percent. You might imagine what the table and balance graph would look like: there would be 0 for the number of women in studies and question marks for the percentage of outcomes related to the disease—there are no numbers to compare.

Since your participation in your care depends on information of benefit and harm, it is hard to imagine how you could decide for, or want, bilateral mastectomies. While there is no information that bilateral mastectomies reduce the already low chances of adverse outcomes for women with DCIS, there is a hint that harm may occur. Cosmetic outcomes are unclear, and second operations to fix the cosmetic outcomes may be needed, so women don't know the consequences from a cosmetic standpoint. A study published 2013 in the *Annals of Surgical Oncology*,[1] for example, found that of 209 women who had bilateral mastectomies, 42 percent had complications, compared with 29 percent of 391 women undergoing unilateral mastectomy (42 percent − 29 percent = 13 percent added chance of harm). Serious complications occurred in 14 percent of bilateral mastectomy patients and only 4 percent of unilateral mastectomy patients (14 percent − 4 percent = 10 percent added chance of harm). These percentages, however, come from an observational study, not an RCT. This study, then, can give us only ballpark numbers.

As an informed decision maker, you now know that there is no trade-off to make for bilateral mastectomy. The benefit side is unknown; the harm side may be 10–13 percent worse but is still uncertain. Hence, at present, if you have DCIS, a physician's recommendation for bilateral mastectomy would be speculative—and speculation has no place in an informing medical profession. Also, while some women feel that removing both breasts may reduce their worry of breast cancer in the future, this statement cannot be made based on evidence. We don't know if women will be better off with bilateral mastectomy, so we don't know if they can or should worry less. Despite the lack of evidence for benefit, bilateral mastectomies for early-stage and other types of breast cancer are on the rise. In 1998, 2 percent of women in California underwent bilateral mastectomy; in 2011, 12 percent did, some of those with DCIS.[2] All three of my patients decided against bilateral mastectomy after learning that no study had been done. Without rigorous study of this option, the treatment should not be proposed to anyone with DCIS.

Story 2

She is a smart, short woman. Her short stature has fueled her desire to succeed against all odds. Some consider her belligerent; I consider her entertaining. We have fun with our differing opinions, and we argue every chance we get. We have an odd relationship for a patient and physician. She commands the time of her visit and tells me in no uncertain terms what she needs and, hence, wants. Everything she reads about medical care is "true," so her "facts" routinely need some adjusting. If she could, she would control every aspect of her life, medical and nonmedical. She has fourteen years of education and is an entrepreneur. She understands physics and engineering and became a successful businessperson, building a business from two employees to over sixty.

On a business trip, she noted blood in her stool, and a colonoscopy performed soon after she returned home showed a large cancer. Surgery was extensive and left her with minor but persistent complications. She had lymph nodes removed at the time of surgery, which showed that the cancer had spread; after surgery, chemotherapy followed. The chemotherapy was difficult on her: the nausea and fatigue kept her from performing her usual duties, and for a while even her business suffered from her absence.

A year after the chemotherapy treatment, a blood test called CEA (carcinoembryonic antigen), ordered on a regular basis to check for early return of cancer, came back positive. Radiology tests showed that the cancer had returned and inhabited a lobe of her liver. Without hesitation, she had one-half of her liver removed. Following this surgery she sought out two opinions from physicians she knew from her business dealings; she asked both if she should have a second round of chemotherapy. These two physicians seemed, on the surface, good choices to offer opinions: they were specialists in cancer of the colon. She was not so sure about taking more chemotherapy, since her cancer had come back despite the first round of chemotherapy.

The opinions from the experts coincided: more chemotherapy would be best. Both physicians concurred, however, that there were no studies to show if more chemotherapy was better. Both physicians were asked what they would do and said they would take more treatment. She did not seek my advice; she would not tell me why. I did not take it personally when she told me she had decided to have more chemotherapy. Her thought was that if she did not do anything more and the cancer came back she would feel that she did not try hard enough. She didn't want to talk more; she was prepared.

She underwent the new treatment and suffered serious chemotherapy toxicity but recovered fully. She used to tell me that studies are not everything; some evidence just makes sense. To her, more chemotherapy made sense. That was five years ago; she is still belligerent to some, and witty to me, and is still leading a thriving business. She looks healthy and happy, and there have been no signs that the cancer has come back: two surgeries, two chemotherapy treatment plans, and no cancer.

Story 3

He is an entrepreneur with a loving wife and well-educated sons. He is, in his own words, "overly healthy" and did not really need to see doctors. However, when he could no longer do "boot camp" workouts with usual vigor, a visit to his physician followed. His anemia was profound. A bone marrow test found cancer in the blood-forming cells. Chemotherapy would halt the cancer, and then a bone marrow transplant would follow.

He did not hesitate to accept the treatment plan, and the first rounds of the chemotherapy treatments did what they were supposed to: cancer cells were dying at a rapid rate—so rapidly, in fact, that his kidney function slowed due to their breakdown products, but then the kidney function recovered. Treatment seemed to be going so well that he and his family thought that perhaps more treatment would be better. They were buoyed by the early good response and wanted more of a good thing. Even though they trusted their treating oncologist fully, they decided to get a "second opinion" about the treatment plan. After all, they had read if the cancer cells were not eliminated completely, the bone marrow transplant might not work as well.

After recovering from the onslaught of the first series of chemotherapy treatments, he and his family traveled to another cancer treatment center. At that visit, he was told he might be better off taking a newer, more aggressive chemotherapy agent in order to "bring the cancer to its knees." The patient and the family did not ask about complications—they thought the side effects could not be worse than those already experienced, which were painful and required frequent trips to the hospital. He assumed the new treatment would be "more of the same." To him, the treatments were doing their work of killing the cancer cells and preparing him for a successful transplant. More had to be better, and he accepted the new treatment wholeheartedly. He came home from the second opinion visit, and his physician added the new agent to the treatment plan. Two weeks later, his liver function slowed. His physician ordered a biopsy of the liver. The examination was never done—the man died of liver failure from toxicity of the new cancer agent.

What Should We Make of These Stories?

Twelve percent of women getting bilateral mastectomies without information that benefit might be possible, and two people chose treatments without knowing what might happen, in one case leading to dire consequences. The latter two patients acted by taking treatments that, in their minds, provided hope and expressed their desire to try their best in difficult situations. Many of us can empathize with these choices. The problem is that these patients could not know how much better the chosen treatments were, and when we don't know if there is benefit, the chance of harm looms while no trade-off is possible.

Being an informed medical decision maker is not easy. Balancing the added chance of benefit against the added chance of harm when comparing tests or treatments is not a simple calculation in your head. In all examples in the preceding chapters, studies had found that one treatment or test versus another reduced the chances of adverse disease outcomes. In other words, some benefit was possible. In these situations, there is a choice to be made based on personal feelings about the chances of good outcomes versus the chances of harmful outcomes.

In other situations, however, good studies may show that the tests or treatments being evaluated provide the same or similar percentages of outcomes. This is another benefit of learning how to participate in your own care—there is no call for a more costly or dangerous test or treatment if it is not better for you. For example, enteric-coated aspirin has been studied and provides no or little benefit over cheaper, plain aspirin. Many blood-pressure-lowering drugs lower blood pressure equally. Having stents placed in arteries may be no better than medicines in some circumstances. Having procedures done to sore knees may be no better than rest and rehabilitation. Many tests provide only redundant information and can be forgone (examples include multiple tests for inflamed pancreas, or to find some causes of low blood counts, or the numerous tests used to diagnose heart ailments). Unilateral mastectomy and conservative surgical treatment of breast cancer provide similar outcomes. Fully participating in your medical decisions will help you know what you do not want, as well as what you do want. In many clinical situations, differing sets of tests or treatments are nearly equal in terms of the outcomes they produce, and knowing of these situations is a great advantage to you.

The stories presented in this chapter reveal a different problem in medical decision making: what do we do if we don't have numbers? There are no easy answers. Some physicians and patients will believe they can "perceive" what is best, but that is wishful thinking. I have two views for you to consider. First, by becoming an informed decision maker and following the process in this book, you will be aware when medical evidence is not good enough to be used. Asking for information about harms and benefits will allow you to know how to act if a choice is to be made, or to not act if no choice is possible. My second comment is this: these wonderful people chose in such a way that their experiences became case reports. We do not know if they made good choices. Also, we don't know if their outcomes are typical and hence can be used to help others who face similar decisions. Evidence from case reports is not helpful for medical decision making (see chapter 7). In situations when you don't know, it may be better for you to become involved in studies. In that way, you will learn more, and your experience will inform others.

18

Clarifications

I believe that your medical care is too important to be left to unopposed opinions of others. Being subjected to critique is the duty of researchers searching for better ways to help us, and of writers who aim to provide a method that allows you to fully participate in your medical decisions. Facing medical decisions side by side with people who have come to me for help has taught me that what I ask of them is difficult, but necessary. In anticipation of some concerns or questions from readers, I offer a few parting thoughts.

Are There Decisions That Patients Should Not Make from an Individual-Only Perspective?

As I mentioned above, some medical care is urgent, and there may be no time for choices. The care of acute, life-threatening illness is ingrained in physicians. The examples in this book have not been about these types of clinical situations. In non-urgent care, with trade-offs for you, you have the time and ability to make informed choices.

I have not yet discussed another situation where there are limits on an individual's ability to make choices. This clinical situation occurs when the outcome of an individual's decision can directly affect the health outcomes of others. For example, it is not our right to decide if we want testing for tuberculosis (TB): if we have TB, treatment is beneficial for us *and* for those who might be exposed to our TB if it is left undetected and untreated. Childhood immunizations such as the MMR vaccine for measles, mumps, and rubella provide benefit not only to our kids but also others' kids. Consider the situation of imposed testing for the HIV virus (human immunodeficiency virus) for blood and tissue donations: infected people may spread the disease via transfusions or transplants, so detection reduces the spread to others. Smoking is a personal choice, but once we learned that being around second-hand smoke was dangerous to others, we passed laws to protect the innocent, removing the smokers' choice to smoke in many public places. These are examples of public health decisions, not of individuals' decisions. The distinction lies in who is potentially affected by the choice via the outcomes suffered—the individual who makes the choice, or others not party to the decision.

Is My Process Too Complex?

Medical decisions can be made in a limited set of ways:

- Physicians, or the medical care system, can make decisions for you with your blessing that they know best. This is a simple way.
- You can make a decision based solely on personal values without knowledge of the consequences, like some of the examples presented. This may be simple too, but it does not allow you to know the percent chances of outcomes you face.
- You can make a decision based solely on percent chances of outcomes. This is relatively simple but does not allow you to include your personal values, as our examples have shown.
- You can make a decision by balancing the trade-off of chances for harm and benefit, based on your personal values, like you have learned in this book.

This last way is not simple. There is nothing simple about making a decision when disease outcomes and test or treatment outcomes compete, and their impacts on your quality of life vary. While the process of informing is straightforward, the balancing of benefit and harm can be gut-wrenching. One way you may be able to simplify this difficult trade-off process is to focus on the most straightforward of the math numbers. If you only know the absolute percent chances of outcomes and can determine differences, you are well on your way to understanding the potential consequences you face. When this becomes second nature to you, count the actual number of people being affected by the different choices out of the entire population of patients studied, like I showed in the CAT example in chapter 8. Last, use the harm:benefit ratio to help you evaluate your feelings about the potential consequences. Even if this process is hard for you, it will be worth your while.

Am I Suggesting Physicians Are Not Needed?

No, physicians are needed. I am only saying that physicians should not decide for you. The best medical decision making occurs with talking, not with tablets, tabloids, or numbers devoid of context. Primary care physicians and nurses should help you determine options, go over harm and benefit numbers, describe what the outcomes entail, and make sure that the people in the studies you are using are like you (remember, for example, the prostate cancer case where the patient's ethnicity was not addressed in clinical studies). I know that some of my patients made choices without their personal physicians, but they did talk with me.

A partnership is best. The following story depicts one idea about how you and your physician can partner to help you make your own medical decisions. A private practicing physician friend of mine proudly and playfully told me that he helped one of his patients come to an informed choice more than I did. (He is always trying to one-up me.) He is not a researcher or trained in evidence-based medicine. His good-natured extolling of his expertise serves as a perfect example of a partnership between a patient, the primary care physician, and me, in this case, as a decision-making consultant. He had referred one of his patients to me, and the patient and I went over her decision. The patient learned the information and could recount numbers exactly. She accurately subtracted outcome differences and began to intuitively make the harm:benefit trade-off.

Her decision involved anticoagulants, or blood thinners. The information I gave her was from an RCT examining the blood thinner she might need. The problem for her was that she did not for certain share the clinical and personal characteristics of the people who were in the study. Her characteristics might increase the chance of harm. I asked her to go back to her physician and make sure that she would fit the population of patients included in the study, as I was not privy to all of her clinical information.

At the end of chapter 7 I listed some potential imperfections with randomized controlled trials (RCTs). There is one more to mention, which is highlighted in a positive way in this example. When patients are recruited for studies, researchers establish criteria for who might be included or excluded from a study. For anticoagulation studies, some patients are too sick, and some have contraindications for anticoagulants because of their higher chance of bleeding. Hence, not all patients will be eligible for the studied options. If a physician applies results of a study to those patients who would have been excluded from the trial in the first place, untoward adverse events may occur. (This would be another example of thinking in terms of populations rather than individuals when making decisions.)

For example, vitamin K antagonists, such as warfarin, are used to reduce adverse events due to clotting of the blood in some patients with cardiovascular disease. Many patients were excluded from the studies of these sorts of blood thinners because they had conditions that increased the risk of bleeding. Prescribing these agents to people who would not be eligible for the study based on exclusion criteria would be inappropriate. In one study, however, researchers found that after the RCTs of these anti-coagulants were published, up to one-quarter of patients in general-care situations who were prescribed these agents had one or more clinical conditions that would have kept them out of any RCT.[1] Most important, 40 percent of people who took these blood thinners and who had bleeding had one or more exclusion criteria; having one exclusion criterion resulted in a nearly threefold increase risk of bleeding, and the risk was higher if more than one exclusion criterion was present. The researchers of the original studies on the blood thinners did a great job of knowing who should not have been in the study, but despite their efforts, the study results were inappropriately applied. This illustrates that some patients should *not* be eligible for some treatments. Being an informed decision maker will help protect you from inappropriately applied options for care.

Back to the story: My physician friend knew of this potential problem because he and I had discussed the issue in the past, and he subsequently told his patient. The new information revealed the harm numbers to be worse, in his patient's eyes, than the potential benefit numbers, and she decided against taking the agent. And that is how he helped one of his patients come to an informed choice: perfect communication, perfect and accurate information for an individual, and a perfect example of how you and your physician can partner for your best care. Information may be shared but, again, not the decision, and my friend's patient made her own choice.

What Might Happen When a Physician Does Not Believe Patients Are the Main Decision Makers?

Medical information is becoming available to all, not just medical practitioners. People will have increasingly more access to useful data on tests and treatments and must know how to use the information to make their choices. But we are in a transition period, and physicians and the business of medicine still think they know best. Hence, sometimes physicians may be challenged by your ability to make your own choice. I do not underestimate what might happen when your knowledge challenges your physician. Some of my patients have told me disturbing stories.

One of my patients was "fired" by her physician (told to find another physician). The patient challenged the data provided by the physician and even brought to the visit the paper the physician was using to make her claims. The data were poor, and the pertinent total number of people in the study was fewer than thirty. When the patient said she was not going to follow the physician's advice, the physician got angry and fired the patient.

Another patient presented a graphic from my blog regarding the shingles vaccine to his physician, and the physician could not interpret the information. Instead, the physician continued to promote the vaccine based on "guidelines."

Another person accompanied her mother to an appointment with her mother's physician to decline an offered surgical intervention based on studies showing no difference in outcomes with surgery. When the daughter showed the study to the physician, the physician said, "My experience trumps any study." To the physician's credit, however, he later recanted his stand and agreed that surgery had little to offer.

This last sentence is an important one: you may face challenge by physicians, but with persistence and an understanding of the information and the trade-offs, most of my patients develop strong partnerships with their physicians. This is ideal, and if you can't do this with your physician, find another.

When There Are Many Studies, Which Do You Use?

It is common that more than one study will exist for the options you are considering. For example, many studies have been done to test aggressive versus usual control for diabetes, like the example in chapter 8 (see figure 1). However, most are not RCT studies, or are not published in journals with high standards for quality (see chapter 19). You may need your physician's help to decide which study is best to use. Also, you can use your critical information skills learned in the apple-a-day example in chapter 7 and 8 to assess the value of the information—if the study is not done well, don't use the information. I use the studies with the largest number of people studied, and the study that examined people who most closely fit the person making the choice. Chapter 19 gives some suggestions for finding the best information.

19

Where to Look for Valuable Medical Information

When I first started practice, finding information was a tedious undertaking. I read textbooks that weighed as much as a baby elephant, or perused medical journals at the library. When I wanted to find a paper about a patient's clinical situation, I either begged the librarian to find it or I went to the library on my own, combed through an index, found the appropriate paper in a journal, walked several floors to where that journal was located, copied the information, and then took it home to read. An afternoon at the library might have netted only a few articles. Times have changed: I now sit at my computer, access an online database (some are suggested below), and follow this straightforward strategy for locating quality medical information:

STRATEGY FOR SEARCHING FOR
MEDICAL INFORMATION
1. Look up a topic area pertinent to the test, treatment, or diagnosis being considered.
2. Cross-reference the topic with the term "randomized controlled trial." The term is a universal search term and is accessed as a cross-reference on the topic.
3. Then cross-reference again, this time with the term "core medical journals" (see below).

This three-step process nets nearly every potentially useful scientific paper that exists on the topic. It usually takes less than two minutes and finds, most often, fewer than twenty studies. A librarian friend and I developed this way to search the literature and learned that following these three steps will find useful information so quickly that we could even use the literature for teaching during daily hospital rounds with patients. Using high-quality literature during the day-to-day care of patients is not the norm, but it should be—it is not possible to remember numbers for every clinical situation, but it is possible to find numbers when you need them.

And times will change even further—if I can find information for your care, so can you. The information you use for your medical care is crucial. The information I used in this book and use with patients comes from the top 100 or so core medical journals out of the nearly 20,000 medical journals total. In fact, in my experience, five networks of journals (the main journals and their specialty offshoots) include many of the best studies: *Lancet, British Medical Journal, Annals of Internal Medicine, New England Journal of Medicine*, and *Journal of the American Medical Association*. The reason that these journals contain the bulk of pertinent studies is that these are the journals most commonly read by physicians and researchers. Hence, these journals are where researchers like to have their work published in order to obtain the largest possible audience. And because they get so many submissions, these journals can choose to publish the studies that are more likely to be good than bad. These journals are a good place to start when seeking the most-likely-true information instead of the more-likely-trumped-up information. But be discerning, as even these journals contain information that may not be true. And surely never expect to learn from newspapers or television; some reports may be good, but you need evidence, not opinions.

Use information from the databases supported by our government that are freely available on the Internet. Those I use most are the National Library of Medicine's MEDLINE, searched via PubMed—http://www.ncbi.nlm.nih.gov/pubmed—and the National Cancer Institute's PDQ, a comprehensive cancer database—http://www.cancer.gov/publications/pdq/. The three-step process outlined above is best used with MEDLINE (and a great way to learn the options for care that have been studied).

I favor these information sources because they give you the best chance at best information. Other sources of information may be of value, but beware—sifting the wheat from the chaff can be harder. I also sometimes use Google to search for information, but when I do I include in my search terms the four letters "PMID" (which stands for PubMed Identifier), which helps the Google search engine find articles from my preferred list of journals. Without these letters in your Google search, you may find information that is more hype than help. Remember, the goal of searching for information is to obtain the numbers that fit you best, not to find out what others think you should do, or buy.

A word of caution: medical papers are tough to read because they are not written for the general public. Also, unfortunately, only abstracted and not full information may be available. The more you become informed about your care and more fully participate in your decisions, the more you will influence how information is presented to you and others like you. The only goal of medical science should be to do accurate studies and make sure you know of the accurate information. At present, however, the articles you read may confuse you because they often obscure the absolute differences in numbers. Don't expect a paper to spring forward with easily understood numbers; it may take some work to obtain the right numbers, so ask your physician for help. I have started a website that shows information used to answer my patients' questions: http://www.sharedmedchoice.com. On the website, I summarize studies and put their useful information in the format shown in this book. The site translates the medical literature's numbers to useful numbers that you can use for your medical decisions.

————

Thank you for joining the journey. Always remember that you matter above all else in your medical decision making. To make that statement a reality rather than just a rallying cry, you must know how to fully participate in your care. Medical care will be best for you only if you are involved in and empowered to make your own choices.

Notes

CHAPTER 3

1 R. A. McNutt, "Shared Medical Decision Making: Problems, Process, Progress," *Journal of the American Medical Association* 292, no. 20 (2004): 2516–18.

2 S. Schwartz and T. Griffin, *Medical Thinking: The Psychology of Medical Judgment and Decision Making* (New York: Springer, 1986), 35–41; D. J. Mazur and D. H. Hickam, "Patients' Interpretations of Probability Terms," *Journal of General Internal Medicine* 6 (1991): 237–40.

3 M. Gladwell, *David and Goliath: Underdogs, Misfits, and the Art of Battling Giants* (New York: Little, Brown, 2013).

4 R. McNutt and N. M. Hadler, "How Clinical Guidelines Can Fail Both Doctors and Patients," *Scientific American Blogs*, November 22, 2013, http://blogs .scientificamerican.com/guest-blog/how-clinical-guidelines-can-fail-both-doctors-and-patients/.

5 "Data by Region," *Dartmouth Atlas of Health Care*, http://www.dartmouthatlas .org/data/region/.

6 B. Lo and M. J. Field, eds., *Conflict of Interest in Medical Research, Education, and Practice* (Washington, D.C.: National Academies Press, 2009), freely available at http://www.ncbi.nlm.nih.gov/books/NBK22942/.

7 T. M. Shaneyfelt and R. M. Centor, "Reassessment of Clinical Practice Guidelines: Go Gently into That Good Night," *Journal of the American Medical Association* 301, no. 8 (2009): 868–69; A. D. Sniderman and C. D. Furberg, "Why Guideline-Making Requires Reform," *Journal of the American Medical Association* 301, no. 4 (2009): 429–31.

8 T. Langer et al., "Conflicts of Interest among Authors of Medical Guidelines: An Analysis of Guidelines Produced by German Specialist Societies," *Deutsches Ärzteblatt International* 109, no. 48 (2012): 836–42, freely available in English at http://www.aerzteblatt.de/int/archive/article?id=132919.

9 N. K. Choudhry et al., "Relationships between Authors of Clinical Practice Guidelines and the Pharmaceutical Industry," *Journal of the American Medical Association* 287, no. 5 (2002): 612–17, freely available at http://jama.jamanetwork .com/article.aspx?articleid=194615.

10 L. A. Hampson et al., "Patients' Views of Financial Conflicts of Interest in Cancer Research Trials," *New England Journal of Medicine* 355 (2006): 2330–37, freely available at http://www.nejm.org/doi/full/10.1056/NEJMsa064160.

11 Hampson et al., "Patients' Views of Financial Conflicts of Interest in Cancer Research Trials."

12 Choudhry et al., "Relationships between Authors of Clinical Practice Guidelines and the Pharmaceutical Industry."

13 L. Lessig, *Republic, Lost*, cited in "Conflict of Interest," *Wikipedia*, December 1, 2015, http://en.wikipedia.org/wiki/Conflict_of_interest.

14 As one example, see P. Thacker, "How an Ethically Challenged Researcher Found a Home at the University of Miami," *Forbes*, September 13, 2011, http://www.forbes.com/sites/paulthacker/2011/09/13/how-an-ethically-challenged-researcher-found-a-home-at-the-university-of-miami/.

15 S. Reardon, "Disclosing Conflicts of Interest Has Unintended Effects," *Nature News*, October 3, 2014, http://www.nature.com/news/disclosing-conflicts-of-interest-has-unintended-effects-1.16077.

16 M. M. Mello, et al., "National Costs of the Medical Liability System," *Health Affairs* 29 (2010): 1569–77, freely available at http://content.healthaffairs.org/content/29/9/1569.long.

17 D. M. Studdert et al., "Defensive Medicine among High-Risk Specialist Physicians in a Volatile Malpractice Environment," *Journal of the American Medical Association* 293, no. 21 (2005): 2609–17, freely available at http://jama.jamanetwork.com/article.aspx?articleid=200994.

CHAPTER 4

1 K. S. Collins, C. Schoen, and D. R. Sandman, *The Commonwealth Fund Survey of Physician Experiences with Managed Care* (New York: The Commonwealth Fund, 1997). Also http://www.ncbi.nlm.nih.gov/pmc/articles/PMC1496869/#b2.

2 S. Jauhar, "Busy Doctors, Wasteful Spending," *New York Times*, July 20, 2014, http://www.nytimes.com/2014/07/21/opinion/busy-doctors-wasteful-spending.html.

3 American College of Physicians, https://www.acponline.org/advocacy/advocacy_in_action/state_of_the_nations_healthcare/assets/2015/summary_of_issues.pdf.

4 M. D. Schwartz, S. Durning, M. Linzer, and K. E. Hauer, "Changes in Medical Students' Views of Internal Medicine Careers from 1990 to 2007," *Archives of Internal Medicine* 8 (2011): 744–49.

5 J. A. Brehaut et al., "Validation of a Decision Regret Scale," *Medical Decision Making* 23 (2003): 281–92.

6 T. Gilovich and V. H. Medvec, "The Experience of Regret: What, When, and Why," *Psychological Review* 102 (1995): 379–95; T. Connolly et al., "Regret and Responsibility in the Evaluation of Decision Outcomes," *Organizational Behavior and Human Decision Processes* 70 (1997): 73–85.

7 Gerald L. Andriole, E. David Crawford et al., "Mortality Results from a Randomized Prostate-Cancer Screening Trial," *New England Journal of Medicine* 360 (2009): 1310–19, freely available at http://www.nejm.org/doi/full/10.1056/NEJMoa0810696.

8 P. A. Ubel et al., "Public Preferences for Prevention versus Cure: What If an Ounce of Prevention Is Worth Only an Ounce of Cure?," *Medical Decision Making* 18 (1998): 141–48.

CHAPTER 5

1 All of these headlines appeared in Medical News Today on November 30, 2012.

CHAPTER 7

1 W. A. Zatonski et al., "Cigarette Smoking, Alcohol, Tea and Coffee Consumption and Pancreatic Cancer Risk: A Case-Control Study from Opole, Poland," *International Journal of Cancer* 53, no. 4 (1993): 601–7.

2 This description is taken from "The Literary Digest," Wikipedia, http://en.wikipedia.org/wiki/The_Literary_Digest (accessed October 16, 2015).

3 A. L. Herbst et al., "Adenocarcinoma of the Vagina—Association of Maternal Stilbestrol Therapy with Tumor Appearance in Young Women," *New England Journal of Medicine* 284 (1971): 878–81, freely available at http://www.nejm.org/doi/full/10.1056/NEJM197104222841604.

4 S. Thaul and D. Hotra, eds., *An Assessment of the NIH Women's Health Initiative* (Washington, D.C.: National Academy Press, 1993), available for download at http://www.nap.edu/catalog/2271/an-assessment-of-the-nih-womens-health-initiative.

5 Thaul and Hotra, *An Assessment of the NIH Women's Health Initiative.*

6 Writing Group for the Women's Health Initiative Investigators, "Risks and Benefits of Estrogen Plus Progestin in Healthy Postmenopausal Women," *Journal of the American Medical Association* 288, no. 3 (2002): 321–33.

CHAPTER 8

1 J. A. Paulos, *Innumeracy: Mathematical Illiteracy and Its Consequences* (New York: Vintage Books, 1990).

2 B. Hemmingsen et al., "Targeting Intensive Glycaemic Control versus Targeting Conventional Glycaemic Control for Type 2 Diabetes Mellitus," *Cochrane Database of Systematic Reviews* 6 (2011): CD008143.

CHAPTER 9

1 D. G. Fryback et al., "The Beaver Dam Health Outcomes Study: Initial Catalog of Health-State Quality Factors," *Medical Decision Making* 13, no. 2 (1993): 89–102.

2 S. J. Cotler et al., "Patient's Values for Health States Associated with Hepatitis C and Physicians' Estimates of Those Values," *American Journal of Gastroenterology* 96 (2001): 2730–36, freely available at http://www.nature.com/ajg/journal/v96/n9/full/ajg2001674a.html.

3 C. J. Ng et al., "A 'Combined Framework' Approach to Developing a Patient Decision Aid: The PANDAs Model," *BMC Health Services Research* 14 (2014): 503, freely available at http://www.biomedcentral.com/1472-6963/14/503.

4 The National Lung Screening Trial Research Team, "Reduced Lung-Cancer Mortality with Low-Dose Computed Tomographic Screening," *New England Journal of Medicine* 365 (2011): 395–409.

CHAPTER 12

1 F. Helgesen, L. Holmberg, J. E. Johansson et al., "Trends in Prostate Cancer Survival in Sweden, 1960 through 1988: Evidence of Increasing Diagnosis of Nonlethal Tumors," *Journal of the National Cancer Institute* 88, no. 17 (1996): 1216–21.

2 G. L. Lu-Yao et al., "Outcomes of Localized Prostate Cancer following Conservative Management," *Journal of the American Medical Association* 302, no. 11 (2009): 1202–9, freely available at http://jama.jamanetwork.com/article.aspx?articleid=184588.

3 M. Djulbegovic et al., "Screening for Prostate Cancer: Systematic Review and Meta-analysis of Randomised Controlled Trials," *British Medical Journal* 341 (2010): c4543, freely available at http://www.bmj.com/content/341/bmj.c4543.long.

4 L. Holmberg et al., "A Randomized Trial Comparing Radical Prostatectomy with Watchful Waiting in Early Prostate Cancer," *New England Journal of Medicine* 347 (2002): 781–89, freely available at http://www.nejm.org/doi/full/10.1056/NEJMoa012794.

5 T. J. Wilt et al., "Radical Prostatectomy versus Observation for Localized Prostate Cancer," *New England Journal of Medicine* 367, no. 3 (2012): 203–13, freely available at http://www.nejm.org/doi/full/10.1056/NEJMoa1113162.

CHAPTER 13

1 M. Alemozaffar et al., "Prediction of Erectile Function following Treatment for Prostate Cancer," *Journal of the American Medical Association* 306, no. 11 (2011): 1205–14, freely available at http://jama.jamanetwork.com/article.aspx?articleid=1104401.

CHAPTER 14

1 T. J. Wilt et al., "Radical Prostatectomy versus Observation for Localized Prostate Cancer," *New England Journal of Medicine* 367, no. 3 (2012): 203–13, freely available at http://www.nejm.org/doi/full/10.1056/NEJMoa1113162.

2 "Prostate Cancer: Screening," U.S. Preventive Services Task Force, May 2012, http://www.uspreventiveservicestaskforce.org/Page/Document/Update SummaryFinal/prostate-cancer-screening.

CHAPTER 15

1 Antithrombotic Trialists' Collaboration et al., "Aspirin in the Primary and Secondary Prevention of Vascular Disease: Collaborative Meta-analysis of

Individual Participant Data from Randomised Trials," *Lancet* 373 (2009): 1849–60, freely available at http://www.thelancet.com/journals/lancet/article/PIIS0140-6736%2809%2960503-1/fulltext.

2 D. L. Bhatt et al., "Clopidogrel and Aspirin versus Aspirin Alone for the Prevention of Atherothrombotic Events," *New England Journal of Medicine* 354, no. 16 (2006): 1706–17, freely available at http://www.nejm.org/doi/full/10.1056/NEJMoa060989.

CHAPTER 16

1 U.S. Preventive Services Task Force, "Screening for Breast Cancer: U.S. Preventive Services Task Force Recommendation Statement," *Annals of Internal Medicine* 151, no. 10 (2009): 716–26, freely available at http://annals.org/article.aspx?articleid=745237.

2 M. Kriege et al., "Efficacy of MRI and Mammography for Breast-Cancer Screening in Women with a Familial or Genetic Predisposition," *New England Journal of Medicine* 351, no. 5 (2004): 427–37, freely available at http://www.nejm.org/doi/full/10.1056/NEJMoa031759.

3 A. B. Miller et al., "Twenty Five Year Follow-up for Breast Cancer Incidence and Mortality of the Canadian National Breast Screening Study: Randomised Screening Trial," *British Medical Journal* 348 (2014): g366, freely available at http://www.bmj.com/content/348/bmj.g366.long.

4 W. A. Berg et al., "Detection of Breast Cancer with Addition of Annual Screening Ultrasound or a Single Screening MRI to Mammography in Women with Elevated Breast Cancer Risk," *Journal of the American Medical Association* 307, no. 13 (2012): 1394–1404, freely available at http://jama.jamanetwork.com/article.aspx?articleid=1148330.

CHAPTER 17

1 M. E. Miller et al., "Operative Risks Associated with Contralateral Prophylactic Mastectomy: A Single Institution Experience," *Annals of Surgical Oncology* 20 (2013): 4113–20.

2 A. W. Kurian et al., "Use of and Mortality after Bilateral Mastectomy Compared with Other Surgical Treatments for Breast Cancer in California, 1998–2011," *Journal of the American Medical Association* 312 (2014): 902–14, freely available at http://jama.jamanetwork.com/article.aspx?articleid=1900512.

CHAPTER 18

1 M. Levi et al., "Bleeding in Patients Receiving Vitamin K Antagonists Who Would Have Been Excluded from Trials on which the Indication for Anticoagulation Was Based," *Blood* 111, no. 9 (2008): 4471–76, freely available at http://www.bloodjournal.org/content/111/9/4471.long?sso-checked=true.

Index

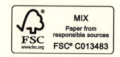